Fact and Prejudice

T0349494

Holm Gero Hümmler • Ulrike Schiesser

Fact and Prejudice

How to Communicate with Esoterics, Fanatics and Conspiracy Believers

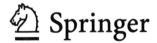 Springer

Holm Gero Hümmler
Bad Homburg, Germany

Ulrike Schiesser
Vienna, Austria

ISBN 978-3-662-66031-7   ISBN 978-3-662-66032-4   (eBook)
https://doi.org/10.1007/978-3-662-66032-4

This book is a translation of the original German edition "Fakt und Vorurteil" by Hümmler, Holm Gero, published by Springer-Verlag GmbH, DE in 2021. The translation was done with the help of artificial intelligence (machine translation by the service DeepL.com). A subsequent human revision was done primarily in terms of content, so that the book will read stylistically differently from a conventional translation. Springer Nature works continuously to further the development of tools for the production of books and on the related technologies to support the authors.

Illustrations by Frances Blüml

This Springer imprint is published by the registered company Springer-Verlag GmbH, DE, part of Springer Nature.
The registered company address is: Heidelberger Platz 3, 14197 Berlin, Germany

Foreword

Holm
Ulrike, what made you decide to write a book with a complete stranger from Germany?

Ulrike
I knew you from skeptics' conferences as the guy who gives lectures on the weirdest conspiracy theories. For me you were inseparably connected with Hitler's UFOs, Nazi fortresses in Antarctica and the "Face on Mars." It wasn't until you asked me if I'd like to write a book with you that I read your books on conspiracy myths and quantum nonsense and saw how long and intensely you've been involved with many topics of pseudoscience. I was very happy about your offer, because my work in the Austrian Bundesstelle für Sektenfragen (Federal Office for Cult Affaires) revolves around exactly these topics: why do people believe irrational things, how does one succeed in changing a worldview, and how do I promote this in conversation? Apart from perhaps the book *Starrköpfe überzeugen* (*Convincing stubborn people*) by Sebastian Herrmann, there are hardly any books that offer concrete help here. So, I thought, "Well, write one yourself."
    How did you come up with the idea to write this book?

Holm
Honestly, I have to say, through the publisher. I didn't want to do it at first. As a natural scientist, how could I write a book on a psychological topic? Then they said, find a co-author, but we want this book – and in retrospect I am very grateful for that. That was before the COVID pandemic, and I didn't expect then that soon, after really every one of my lectures, I would be

confronted with the question: "But what do I do when my uncle talks non-sense?" And that is indeed not an easy question.

I have the impression that you can find a lot of things online and in books that are supposed to help you – but these are mostly argumentation guides from philosophy, which first assume that the other side has any interest at all in a factual, substantive discussion. Some of the recommendations that one comes across in this way also seem quite manipulative to me. If I were on the opposite side and, for example, someone constantly asked me to justify my position by asking questions, but was not prepared to take a stand himself, then I would very quickly break off the conversation.

Ulrike

I am also often asked for a recipe, a trick to get someone to see the error of their ways, to turn their worldview upside down, and to behave in a way that the inquirer thinks is right. This is usually well-intentioned, and there is some-times pure desperation and frustration behind the request, but it doesn't work that way. People are complex and not so easily manipulated into a direction they don't want to go. My wish with this book was to build up a buffet of dif-ferent suggestions and ideas for self-service, to give food for thought. Most important to me, however, are not the methods, but the attitude with which I communicate. We need more understanding and mutual respect instead of outrage and denigration.

Holm

At the same time, especially in the environment of right-wing extremist con-spiracy myths, I repeatedly come across statements where one can only be outraged – or at least has to draw a clear line. So it really is not easy.

So how do you approach a topic where there can be so many and some-times contradictory answers? We decided to talk to very different people who have a lot of experience in such discussions, on social networks, in blogs, in the comment columns of newspapers, or quite directly, in the doctor's office or in youth work. But it was especially important for us to talk to people who have been on the other side themselves, who believed in conspiracy myths, alternative medicine, or ghosts, but then fundamentally changed their world-view. What made a vaccine-critical mother change her mind, what made a YouTube guru, a homeopathic doctor or a conspiracy believer change theirs? And what can we learn from this for discussions with such people?

Ulrike

In my field of work, the direct care and therapy of people who have been harmed by gurus and charlatans, there are only a few experts, and it is easy to feel a little lonely. This made the input from the interviews with people who also work in their professional field with issues such as extremism, superstition, anti-science, and toxic spirituality all the more enjoyable for me. It was interesting how often we had similar experiences and represented similar approaches. And then there was the small group of researchers who approach the topic with the tools of science.

Holm

Just being able to interview all of these insanely exciting people was worth writing this book, and it's a bit of a shame that we couldn't just quote a lot more from the interviews. But it was supposed to be a book that would help you very directly in discussions. So, we had to structure it a bit more.

In the first part, we bring some order to the problems one faces in such a discussion. What psychological effects are at work when we (yes, all of us!) believe nonsensical things? What could we learn about the process of changing one's mind from the interviewees who were once on the other side? What are the options for approaching a discussion? There are more than you might think. What role do the situation and your relationship to the otherside play? What can and do you realistically want to achieve in a discussion?

Ulrike

In the second part, we go through different situations in which conflicts can typically arise. Depending on whether the conversation is with my grandpa, my boss, my midwife, my 8-year-old nephew or in a discussion forum on the Internet, there are different recommendations. The third part is a collection and summary of the most important tips, but also an argumentation aid for frequently used phrases.

Holm

The fact that this book actually came about and that we wrote it together is largely thanks to Alexander Waschkau from the Hoaxilla Podcast. He, a psychologist himself, was the first person from the skeptical environment I talked to about the project, and it was he who said, "Why don't you talk to Ulrike?" Even though the two of them were not among our actual interview partners, ideas from my conversations with Alexander and Alexa Waschkau have also been incorporated into the book in many places. I am also grateful to my partner Theresa, who not only accompanied the writing process with patience and understanding, but also provided many insights into the world of thought of the "other side."

Ulrike

Thanks to our patient and competent contacts at Springer-Verlag, Lisa Edelhäuser and Carola Lerch, and to our wonderful illustrator Frances Blüml, who conjured vivid images out of complex content! Thanks to all the people who have given me important insights and perspectives in conversations, whether as interview partners for this book, clients, or colleagues, especially the colleagues of the Bundesstelle für Sektenfragen German Müller and Sylvia Neuberger. Thanks to my test and proofreaders Wolfgang and Irmi Suntinger, Ingrid Mayer, Michael Mikas, and Stefano Falchetto. To Günter Mandl and Blake Sclanders, my writing hosts. To Stefan, Timon, and Kilian, who have tolerated this book as a time-consuming adopted child in the family.

About the Interview Partners

This book would not have been possible without the interview partners who shared their knowledge and experiences with us. Some of them have regular professional or volunteer experience with discussions of the kind considered here; others were once believers themselves and have told us about their own transformation processes. In part, their stories are briefly presented in Chap. 3; in part, they are quoted at various points in the book. In many places, their experiences and assessments have been incorporated into the text. We would like to thank all the interview partners and introduce them briefly below.

Florian Aigner
The physicist Florian Aigner is responsible for science communication at the Vienna University of Technology. Active in the skeptic scene for years, he is the author of two non-fiction books on the basics of scientific thinking, a science blogger and columnist. In his work, he regularly participates in online discussions with believers, appears in the media and speaks at events.

Florian Albrecht
Physician Florian Albrecht has incorporated alternative medicine methods into his work in various positions. After a fundamental change of mind, he is now established as a family doctor and vigorously advocates a strictly science-based medicine in his work and beyond. After being active in the skeptic scene for some time, he has since distanced himself and considers large parts of the organized skeptics to be half-hearted and inconsistent.

Sebastian Bartoschek

The psychologist Sebastian Bartoschek researched conspiracy beliefs in his doctoral thesis and was simultaneously active for many years as a journalist and author. In doing so, he repeatedly interviewed prominent esotericists and conspiracy believers such as Erich von Däniken or Axel Stoll. In the meantime, he has his own company as his main occupation, which mainly offers expert assessments and diagnostic expertise.

Lydia Benecke

Psychologist Lydia Benecke has been working with sex offenders and violent criminals for years and advises police and media on criminal psychology issues. She has written several books on crime and mental disorders and is active against right-wing extremism, for scientific education and the rights of discriminated social groups. In the process, she has been the target of aggressive campaigns by right-wing extremists and conspiracy believers on several occasions.

Susan Blackmore

Psychologist Susan Blackmore has spent many years in research on parapsychology and paranormal experiences. After initially approaching the topic as a firm believer, in the course of her own work she became more critical and finally an active skeptic. Later, she quit active parapsychological research, became active for humanism and wrote several books on the concept of memes, ideas that reproduce and evolve similar to genes.

Thomas F.

Thomas F. is a pediatrician who works in a hospital, where he is primarily involved in the intensive care of newborns. During his studies he was convinced of the effectiveness of homeopathy and was a member of a corresponding working group. In the course of his professional career he became aware of the ineffectiveness of this method. In the meantime, he has become a committed advocate of science-based medicine and attaches great importance to providing appropriate advice to the parents of the children he cares for.

Krista Federspiel

Medical journalist and author Krista Federspiel has been one of the most vocal critics of alternative medicine and esotericism in Austria for decades. In the wake of her retirement, she has withdrawn from the forefront of skeptical activism, but maintains a presence and reports on her many years of experience in discussions with believers, the media, and politics. In 2020, she was awarded the "Austrian Cross of Honor for Science and Art" for her commitment.

Christopher French

Chris French is a professor of psychology at Goldsmiths College of the University of London and head of the anomalistic psychology research department. His most important areas of research are the belief in paranormal phenomena and the psychology of unusual experiences, on which he himself has turned from a believer to a skeptic. As part of his research he also regularly tests people who believe they have supernatural abilities.

Natalie Grams

Natalie Grams, a physician, had her own private homeopathic practice for several years until, in the course of research for her own book, she realized the pharmaceutical ineffectiveness of homeopathy. As a result, she gave up her practice and became the figurehead of German homeopathy critics. She was repeatedly subjected to fierce, even personal attacks by her former colleagues. After several career changes, she took up employment at the German agency for disease control and prevention in early 2021.

Bernd Harder

Bernd Harder is a journalist and has been active in the skeptic organization Gesellschaft zur wissenschaftlichen Untersuchung von Parawissenschaften (GWUP) since the 1990s. At the same time, he has written numerous books on skeptical topics, especially in the field of popular culture. As the person in charge of the GWUP's blog, he regularly has to intervene in the blog's commentary discussions as a moderator. He also has discussions about science and belief systems in connection with his lectures and readings, and in projects at schools.

Britt Marie Hermes

American Britt Marie Hermes has a degree as a naturopath and worked for 3 years in an alternative medicine cancer clinic. She then turned her back on alternative medicine and began publicly denouncing the dangers of such practices. When she was sued by an American natural healer because of a critical article in her blog, she received a lot of support, including financial help, from the international skeptic scene. She now lives in Kiel and is doing her doctorate on the genetics of microorganisms.

Lisa L.

Lisa L. grew up in a family of followers of Jehovah's Witnesses. As a child, she was firmly integrated into the faith community, but later developed increasing doubts about the faith and, as a young adult, managed to break away from Jehovah's Witnesses with the help of her older sisters. She is now studying and supporting other dropouts.

Christian Lübbers

Ear, nose, and throat specialist Christian Lübbers gained national notoriety in 2017 when he had to remove homeopathic globules from the ear of a 4-year-old child. As a leading figure of the Informationsnetzwerk Homöopathie (INH), he is one of the most prominent critics of homeopathy in Germany and established the term #Globukalypse for the decline of the belief in homeopathy in Germany, especially via Twitter.

Sophie Niedenzu

Molecular biologist and publicist Sophie Niedenzu worked for more than 8 years as a journalist specializing in science, education, and medicine and in community management for the Austrian daily newspaper Der Standard. There she moderated, among other things, the discussion forums of the online edition. Later, she worked as an editor for a medical publisher. She currently works in the public relations department of the Austrian Medical Association, where her responsibilities include health policy reporting in the affiliated journal.

Andreas Peham

Andreas Peham is a political scientist specializing in research on right-wing extremism and anti-Semitism and works for the Documentation Center of Austrian Resistance in Vienna. He has written books and contributed to anthologies on the far-right scene in Austria and beyond, and regularly appears in the media as an expert on these topics. Especially in political education in schools, he regularly experiences discussions with students who are inclined towards conspiracy beliefs or political extremism.

Martin Puntigam

The comedian and actor Martin Puntigam has been on stage for more than 30 years and has always been committed to the communication of science. He is widely known as the central figure of the science comedy group Science Busters, which brought this innovative means of science communication to unprecedented impact in Austria.

Fabian Reicher
Social worker Fabian Reicher is active for the Austrian Extremism Information Centre in the field of supporting distancing and exits from extremist groups. His areas of work include both right-wing extremism and jihadism. In his work, he is regularly in direct dialogue with radicalized or at-risk youth. He is the coordinator of the project *Jamal al-Khatib – My Way!*, a multi-professional, participatory peer-to-peer online film project with the goal of countering Islamist propaganda with alternative narratives from young people who have left the jihadist scene.

Jessica Schab
Jessica Schab made a name for herself as a young woman with spiritual messages in YouTube videos. Within a very short time, she amassed a following of over one million subscribers. Confronted with her own responsibility for her followers, she turned away from esotericism, tried to support others in leaving and is currently involved in the documentary "Confessions of a Former Guru" about her own story.

Theresa Stange
Theresa Stange became a mother at the age of 19 and was a convinced opponent of vaccination for several years. Critical of the alternative medical procedures often recommended within that scene, she remained uncertain for years, always seeking validation for her opposition to vaccinations. Finally, it was only after separating from the father of her two children and with a new partner that she found the confidence to make up the missed vaccinations.

Hayley Stevens
Hayley Stevens was the organizer of a British ghost hunting group at the age of 16 and then became a prominent critic of the ghost believer scene. After prolonged activity in the British skeptic environment, the psychology student has since distanced herself from the skeptic scene, which she perceives as contemptuous of believers and in parts misogynistic. Still, she continues to actively advocate enlightenment and scientific thinking.

Stephanie Wittschier
Stephanie Wittschier was a conspiracy believer for many years, which caused considerable tension within her family. After she found her way out of the scene, she and her husband founded the Facebook group "Nothing but the Truth" and the page "The Loose Screw," which provide cuttingly humorous education about conspiracy myths.

Contents

List of Figures

Part I

Basics

Ultimately, this book is intended to be a kind of guidebook that provides practical food for thought and ideas for discussions between fact and prejudice. First, however, we need to address a few very basic questions. In the purely fictional but quite common story of a young woman, we look at the situations in which we encounter such discussions and how helpless we can be in them, even if we actually have good arguments. We can't get past the question of why people believe in conspiracies, ghosts, or miracle cures. We can anticipate part of the punchline to this right away: It has a lot to do with the fact that we all like to believe such things, and that we find it very challenging to be dissuaded from what we believe. Anyone who tries to persuade other people away from esotericism, fanaticism or conspiracy beliefs is fighting against a whole arsenal of psychological mechanisms that actually serve above all to make our lives easier. Nevertheless, there are always people who manage to break away from such belief systems. We will illustrate this by looking at the stories of well-known and less well-known people who have talked to us about their experiences in changing their minds. Of course, the question of what role conversations with scientifically minded people played in this process is particularly exciting. Finally, we look at what basic possibilities there are for approaching these conversations – and there are more than one might think, just as such a conversation can take place under very different conditions. The goal cannot and does not always have to be to convince the other side. Accepting this can save you a lot of frustration.

1

Introduction

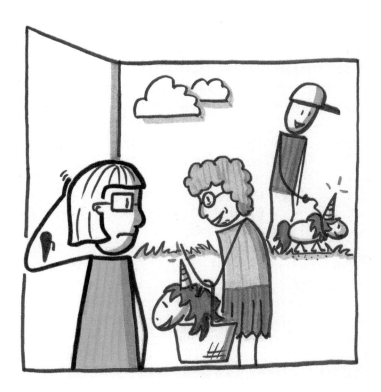

H. G. Hümmler, U. Schiesser, *Fact and Prejudice*,
https://doi.org/10.1007/978-3-662-66032-4_1

"You just can't argue with Globeheads."

Sophie is dismayed. Five minutes ago, she had no idea what a globehead was, and now she's one herself – and she's quite sure of it. Yet it all started out quite harmlessly.

Actually, she just wanted to present a few vacation photos from the first sailing trip she took with her children. In the Facebook group where she shared the pictures, there are mainly people who share her love for the Baltic Sea, who can name every lighthouse, every striking piece of coastline in the pictures. For the more well-known places, someone actually always has their own vacation memories to contribute. People give advice on how child-friendly the campsite in Heiligenhafen is and what to do on Usedom in bad weather. Krischan, who rides his motorcycle to Fehmarn every free weekend and whom Sophie and her husband are keen to meet in person, regularly reports on the weather on the island and on the atmosphere in the restaurants.

The administrators of the group rarely intervene in the conversations. There is a harmonious, family atmosphere among the regular participants. They agree that the Storebælt Bridge is a magnificent structure, but that a bridge across the Fehmarn Belt would be a crime. Some swear by the Danish island of Lolland for their vacations; others find neighboring Falster more beautiful. Occasionally there are discussions about whether Timmendorf is really over-priced or whether Kühlungsborn is not actually much more overpriced. As a rule, however, people quickly agree again – the main thing is that they don't go to the North Sea.

So Sophie didn't think anything of it at first when, in response to a picture of the chalk cliffs on the island of Rügen, the question arose as to whether Bornholm, which is about 100 km away, could be seen from Rügen. After all, the Alps are similarly far away from Munich and are easily visible in good weather. With her scientific education and her experience in navigation while sailing, she was able to quickly calculate that from the highest point on Rügen, the 161 m high Piekberg, one should be able to see the equally high Rytterknægten on Bornholm in good visibility. From the chalk cliffs, however, Bornholm should be completely hidden behind the horizon under normal atmospheric conditions. In a comment to the picture she briefly described the result and the basic idea of the calculation. She did not expect any contradiction. Occasionally in such a calculation someone does not understand that refraction of light in the atmosphere increases visibility under normal conditions, but she would have been prepared to explain that. What she didn't expect was the comment, "You actually believe that shit, right?" "What do you mean? What shit?" she inquired, half unsure, half annoyed. "Well, the nonsense about that globe. That the earth is a sphere with a circumference of 44,000 km and all that."

Klaus, from whom the aggressive interjection came, has not been in the group for long. He occasionally attracts attention with odd comments, but is otherwise an asset with his profound knowledge of the geography and history of the Baltic coast of Mecklenburg. His views may be strange, and Sophie has long felt that discussing politics with him would not be a good idea, but he is definitely not stupid.

Sophie has never met a person who seriously claims that the earth is flat. Her first thought was that someone was probably making fun of her. In a group of people she only knows from her online profile, but many of whom she considers friends, she doesn't want to embarrass herself or risk a pointless argument. So she made a conscious effort to be factual in her initial responses. She explained her calculations once again, but, as Klaus immediately noted, on the basis of what he considered the completely absurd assumption that the earth is a sphere. Her remark that navigation in seafaring has been based on the curvature of the earth for centuries, if not millennia, impresses him just as little as her remark that at the sea the curvature of the earth can be seen easily with binoculars after all.

"Have you ever seen anywhere that the horizon is curved???"

The nature of the question seems so absurd to Sophie that she doesn't even want to respond to it.

"That's what you see, isn't it, that a ship moving away disappears behind the curvature of the earth?"

"You believe that because you've been talked into it. It just looks that way because of the perspective."

"Klaus, that's nonsense!"

"You just can't argue with Globeheads."

A few seconds later, Klaus links to an image with a straight horizon and a superimposed commentary about the stupidity of globe believers who have been persuaded that they are seeing a sphere when water surfaces are visibly flat. The image comes from a Facebook page on which similar depictions of the flat earth alternate with climate change denial, mockery of the allegedly fake moon landing, creationism and anti-Semitic agitation.

Sophie is stunned, horrified and captivated at the same time. Like a bystander who can't tear her gaze away from a particularly bloody accident, she clicks through more and more new images, articles and videos and the comments on them for over an hour. The arguments put forward as to why the earth cannot be a sphere seem almost touchingly naive to Sophie: it looks flat from the ground, so it is flat. Depictions of the southern hemisphere show people standing on their heads, asking why they don't fall off the earth. The page has 4000 fans, and judging by the unanimity of the comments, apparently most of them actually believe in a flat Earth. After a brief search, Sophie comes across half a dozen other pages and discussion groups of similar content, all with thousands of followers. Finally, she can't hold back any longer, trying in her own comments to at least point out the most absurd errors in thinking. After 5 min, other readers ridicule her as a sleep sheep. After 10 min, she can no longer comment on the site: One of the administrators has blocked her.

Over the next few days, Sophie is repeatedly annoyed that she got involved in such a pointless discussion in the first place and even ended up leaving comments on the Flat Earth page under her real name. Perhaps Klaus and his friends from this site are now laughing their heads off that she actually fell for their crude satire.

* * *

Between family and work, Sophie actually has neither the time nor the nerve to get caught up in pointless, annoying discussions. She is proud of the efficiency and single-mindedness with which she has managed to get back into work after her maternity leave and has even managed to secure a management position in her company on a part-time basis. In addition to the three employees from other functions who are temporarily seconded to her small team, she is now to hire someone herself for the first time. Over the past few weeks, she has read various articles on team composition and personnel selection, created a detailed requirements profile and coordinated it with the personnel manager, worked through folders full of resumes, and finally conducted interviews and observed the applicants in role plays and while solving case studies. Selecting her first permanent employee will be the most important decision in her professional life so far, and as uncertain as such a decision inevitably is, she at least doesn't want to make any obvious mistakes.

Sophie somehow imagined this decision to be easier. As well prepared as she has been, even after the interviews and case studies she finds it incredibly difficult to assess which of the applicants would be best suited for the job or even who she could work well with in the long term. In a way, she finds it a relief that Mr. Fischer, the company's longtime personnel manager, is involved in the selection process. With his patriarchal demeanor, rumbling voice and always somewhat intrusive sense of humor, Mr. Fischer seems a bit of a dinosaur in the company's young management ranks. Among colleagues, it is said that he is still in his position primarily because he "keeps the labor union folks under control". His unshakable confidence in his own judgment fills Sophie with a kind of comforting resignation: as long as he agrees with the new hire, she may not have found the most suitable employee, but in any case she will never have to justify her decision.

The decisive meeting, which is to propose the final candidate to the management, is attended by her three coworkers, each of whom has only participated in the interviews with individual candidates, as well as Mr. Fischer, who has only spoken briefly, but with all the applicants. Sophie first presents her evaluation grid, which she has drawn up according to the requirements profile and according to which she has already evaluated the candidates for herself. Mr. Fischer's comment that one must also take into account the likelihood of an offer being accepted convinces her. She is shocked by his next comment, however:

"We also have to take the graphological assessment into account."

"A graphological assessment?"

"Yes. The results for all candidates have been available since Friday. That always goes very quickly."

"Yes, but – why?"

"We have graphological assessments done for all candidates for management positions. We've always done it that way."

"That's not very meaningful."

"It was no different with you back then."

"But I didn't give you a handwriting sample."

"The signature is enough for that."

Sophie lets it go for the moment. She is sure that an applicant's handwriting is not a suitable tool for personnel selection, but without preparation she simply lacks solid arguments to engage in a discussion with an experienced HR manager. Reluctantly, she adds the column in the evaluation grid – determined to enforce the lowest possible weighting for it later.

Then she presents her own assessments of the applicants according to the evaluation grid. For Sophie, two clear favorites emerge, although she tries to be aware of her subjective sympathies and to hold them back: One of her favorites is also a mother and is looking to start her career again after a long break for parenting, right away with a full-time position. She is highly qualified and has relevant experience, presents herself as very adaptable except for the obvious limits in working hours because of the children, perhaps sold herself a bit too modestly and reservedly in the interviews. Virtually tied in Sophie's rating is a young man, very dedicated, with excellent degrees, who excelled in the case studies and role plays despite his lack of work experience.

The members of Sophie's team, with whom she has deliberately not talked about this topic beforehand, take good note of her evaluations, but before the coffee break, Mr. Fischer absolutely has to present his view of things, including the graphological reports. The young man rated well by Sophie is a careerist and a phony, they say, and the highly qualified mother is not a team player and is emotionally unstable. Mr. Fischer obviously favors another applicant, a man with professional experience, but in a somewhat different subject area. In the case studies, he has been dominant and self-centered. In Sophie's estimation, he would be a good candidate for other roles in the company, but not for her team.

While the others drink their coffee, Sophie sits down at her computer, searching for information on graphology. In just 10 minutes, she has what she needs: an article from a portal about pseudoscience, a scathing assessment by a renowned professor of business psychology and, from the sources given there, two scientific studies. The results are clear: Instead of selecting employees according to graphological assessments, you might as well roll the dice.

Mr. Fischer acknowledges the scientific results with a very simple statement: He has been in the business for 20 years and has always had good experiences with graphological assessments. Above all, unlike in a job interview, one cannot pretend with one's handwriting. After all, without the reports, they wouldn't even have come up with the idea of discussing whether Sophie's favorites were careerists or emotionally unstable. Sophie's objection that there was no reason whatsoever that they should be had no effect.

In the end, Sophie does exactly what she actually wanted to avoid and concentrates on preventing Mr. Fischer's favorite. After a lengthy discussion, they agree on the young man from Sophie's suggestions. She is happy to take the assumed risk that he might be a careerist and a phony.

In the evening, after her daughter is in bed, Sophie researches the scientific evaluation of graphology again for hours. In the end, she has a complete binder full of articles and studies, and the results don't get any more flattering for graphology. She can clearly prove that it is a pseudoscientific concept. During the following sleepless night, Sophie considers whether she should try to talk to Mr. Fischer again without any specific reason, or whether she should protest directly to the management against the use of graphological reports. When she finally falls asleep, she knows she will do neither. The facts are clear, but the discussion is pointless.

* * *

"Charlotte and Philipp banged their heads together on the slide. Should I give her arnica, too?"

"Arnica?" Sophie casually answers the message on her smartphone at a red light while on her way from work to the playground, where her friend Steffi is waiting for her with the kids.

"Well, homeopathic globules."

"NO!"

"All right, I know you don't take anything like that. I just thought, because she cries so much. So, see you in a bit, we'll wait for you."

"THANK YOU!"

By the time Sophie is back at a red light and able to write that final response, agonizing minutes have passed, and she's only a few hundred yards from the playground. She is distinctly uncomfortable with the situation. Actually, she is annoyed by Steffi's suggestion to give her daughter Charlotte pseudo-medicine. On the other hand, she is incredibly grateful that Steffi stepped in so easily and took Charlotte from kindergarten, as she has done so many times before, when Sophie had to stay longer at the company because of the hiring of the new employee. Sophie constantly struggles with the feeling that she has far too few opportunities to return the favor to Steffi.

The situation doesn't get any easier when she arrives at the playground: "Mom, Philipp got those little sweet balls, and he doesn't have a bump at all!"

Sophie picks up her daughter, which is starting to become an effort with Charlotte now almost 6 years old.

"Let me see, little angel. Where did you bump into each other?"

"On the slide."

"No, where on your head? There on the side? That doesn't look so bad. We'll put an ice pack on it later at grandma's, and it'll be gone in a few days. Do you feel sick?"

"No, but it hurts!!!" Charlotte bursts into tears.

"Hi, Sophie, I'm sorry." Steffi looks at her in dismay. "The two of them slid behind each other, and Philipp couldn't get away in time. I couldn't get there fast enough either."

"Don't worry about it. This kind of thing happens to them all the time. I'm so grateful you were able to step in and pick her up again."

"No problem. We were going to the playground anyway."

"Mom, I want those little balls too. I have a really bad bump, and it hurts!" interjects Charlotte.

"Angel, we don't need that. Later, at grandma's, we'll put something cold on it, and then it will quickly get better. Look, Philipp has built a sand castle, don't you want to play there?"

Steffi looks at her apologetically: "Hey, I had to give Philipp something earlier. I don't know how else to get him calm when he's hurt so badly. And arnica works really well for him. Maybe you should try it."

"I don't have to try anything, Steffi. It's already been tried in umpteen studies on thousands of people. And there's no active ingredient in it. It's just sugar."

"I don't know why. It just helps with Philipp."

"I just don't want Charlotte to learn that you have to take something every time something is wrong. She doesn't understand that it's just a placebo. Couldn't you have just given them both some gummy bears?"

"I don't take candy to the playground!"

"But sugar balls. Sorry, I'm stressed today. Do you give him stuff like that when he's acting up?"

"Of course not. You can't sedate children with medication. I mean, the first few weeks in kindergarten he got Pulsatilla, for separation anxiety. The pediatrician recommended it."

"Steffi, you should give Philipp Zappelin," Sophie hears from the picnic table behind the slide. "That's also homeopathic and has nothing to do with sedating, but then he's not so hyperactive, doesn't terrorize the others all the time, and doesn't hurt himself as often. And of course my Johannes always gets Arnica D12 when he has hurt himself so badly. Then he doesn't get such a bump like poor Charlotte."

Sophie would have gladly done without the interference of Nadine, against whose son the suddenly recovered Charlotte and Philipp are currently defending Philipp's sand castle with their combined forces. Only now does she notice that two other parents at the picnic table have overheard the conversation. To be on the safe side, she swallows the snippy answer that the cheeky Nadine could well have taken and goes on the defensive:

"She doesn't usually get bumps like that either. Not even without homeopathy."

"You really shouldn't be so opinionated, though." Nadine has no intention of letting Sophie off the hook so easily. "It doesn't matter why homeopathy helps. In any case, it helps without chemistry."

"Nadine, everything is chemistry." Sophie imagines drawing the structural formula of sugar in the sand of the play area.

"Homeopathy is natural, though. But if it's not from big pharma, of course it's not going to help you. Just because the scientists haven't understood it yet. They don't know everything either. There are just more things between heaven and earth … He who heals is right."

"It is very well researched how homeopathy works: not beyond the placebo effect."

"Yeah, sure, we're all imagining it. After all, we're all stupid. But it also works on our little one, and he's only seven months old. It even helped in the first week when he cried so much. He got globules from the midwife. And they also help with our cat. Even the vet recommended it."

"Nadine, the placebo effect has nothing to do with imagination, and yes, there is a placebo effect with babies and animals, too. Let's talk about it another time, okay? Charlotte needs some rest right now, I think."

"It's okay. Believe what you want. Take care, and say hello to your husband for us."

As Sophie thanks Steffi once again and leaves the playground with Charlotte, she sees the silent looks of the other parents directed at her. Charlotte, somewhat intimidated, takes her mother's hand, probably wondering if she is to blame for the tense tone between the adults.

"Come on, Charlotte, you know what we're going to do now? We're going to stop at the ice cream parlor on the way to Grandma's house. That's going to stop your head from hurting. I need completely different sweet little balls now: Raspberry, vanilla and chocolate."

Escaping from the unpleasant discussion, at the exit of the playground, Sophie looks with some relief into the grinning face of Erik, whose daughter Sina is also in Charlotte's kindergarten group. Erik is a dad with heart and soul and a remarkable amount of time on his hands, who always has a big bag of fruit with him on the playground and is happy to share – and occasionally Sophie gets the impression that he's flirting with her a little.

"Hello Charlotte, hello Sophie. Come on, don't look like that. Don't let them drive you crazy. Of course it's nonsense. Ten kinds of globules are supposed to help against everything, and for everyone. It's obvious that this can't work. The best thing is to add Bach's Rescue Remedy on top of it, that's expected to help against everything. But you should really go to my uncle; he is a professional alternative practitioner, he can put together exactly the right active ingredients and the appropriate potencies for the most common problems for Charlotte. Children in particular need very individual homeopathic ingredients and potencies. He does it scientifically, with a technical device, with bioresonance."

*   *   *

"Mom, what kind of book is that?"

The paperback with the strange promises about the supposedly forbidden healing of all kinds of diseases, which Sophie has found on the coffee table while her mother drags a huge bowl of cookies for Charlotte from the kitchen, does not inspire much confidence in her.

"I got this from Horst, from the running club. Because of my arthritis. The man who wrote it also had arthritis once. He's quite an impressive person."

Sophie briefly flips through the book.

"Mom, it's about this MMS, this supposed miracle stuff, I read about it. It's dangerous!"

"Anyway, it helped this man, and he had really bad arthritis. No doctor could help him. And now it's gone. And it also helped Horst with his shingles. And it's supposed to protect against dementia, too."

"Mom, you're not taking this MMS too, are you?"

"Sophie, sweetheart, I don't take MMS. It's got acid in it, and you know I have such a weak stomach."

"All right, Mom. Promise me you won't start taking it either!"

"The one I take is much more harmless. It's called chloroxi … wait a minute, here it is in the book. Chlorine dioxide. Horst ordered it from the Internet. The pharmacy doesn't have it."

"That will have its reasons."

While Sophie starts searching for information in her smartphone, her mother, visibly relieved, turns her attention to Charlotte and the ancient toy grocer's shop that has been waiting for grandchildren in her basement for the last 30 years. Sophie can't stay quiet for long while reading, though:

"Mom, this chlorine dioxide is exactly the same thing you take in MMS, only without citric acid – and that's guaranteed to be the only thing about it that isn't harmful. How can you take such toxic stuff?"

"It helps me. And Horst says he doesn't even need pills for blood pressure anymore."

"Mom, you're not going to stop taking your blood pressure medicine! Your grandkids would like to have a few more years of you."

"It's okay, honey, but really, my ankles hurt a lot less already."

"MMS. Miracle Mineral Supplement. They're already calling it miracle mineral supplement. How can you swallow something like that? Tell me, are you out of your mind? This is a disinfectant. It's like pouring toilet cleaner down your throat."

"Yes, exactly. That's what Horst explained to me. It kills all the bad bacteria in the intestines. Because they perforate the intestine, and then they're in the blood, and then you get arthritis. And shingles. And blood pressure. And maybe cancer, too."

"Mom, if you have holes in your intestines, you need emergency surgery, like your nephew did when he had his appendix burst. Otherwise you're dead. And bacteria in the intestines is what we need, otherwise we can't digest our food."

"After all, that only kills the harmful bacteria, the acidic ones. It doesn't do anything at all to the alkaline ones that we need. And neither to humans for that matter."

"Did Horst tell you that, too? And you think he knows more about it than your family doctor and your rheumatologist and everyone at the pharmacy?"

"But you can see that it works. And Horst reads about it all the time on the Internet. And he has books by famous doctors who all recommend chlorine dioxide, too. But you obviously know everything better and you're not a doctor either."

"It says here that the Federal Institute for Drugs and Medical Devices has banned its sale as a drug. And they have lots of highly qualified medical doctors and pharmacists, and they get advice from the best scientists. And there's one guy who's been sentenced to three years in prison for selling this."

"Yeah, that's in the book, too. That's all because the chlorine dioxide just helps so well and is so well proven and much cheaper than all the chemistry from pharma. That's why they're making sure it's banned, because otherwise they won't sell anything anymore."

* * *

Actually, Sophie, the fictional protagonist of our introduction, has the better arguments in all these discussions. She has good background knowledge, she doesn't argue rashly, and when it comes to topics she's not familiar with, she informs herself from well-founded sources. Nevertheless, her argumentation always comes to nothing. She takes her opponent seriously and tries to remain factual for as long as possible and not to provoke unnecessarily. Even in confrontation, she tries as hard as she can in the emotional situation to find common ground so that she can still get her content across. And every time, her content is simply pushed aside, and her counterparts insists on their demonstrably factually incorrect position.

Many a skeptical-scientifically thinking person who has already faced similar situations will have thought to himself that in one or the other of the four situations presented, any argumentation is simply pointless, that one cannot win either way and that it is best not to get involved in a discussion at all. In reality, however, such detachment is often not possible.

If, as in the example of the flat earth discussion, one is dealing with a more or less anonymous person on the Internet, then one actually has the option of simply turning off the computer and ignoring objectively false assertions – in most cases, anyway. If such claims are likely to damage one's own reputation, for example because they give the impression that one agrees with them or has no counterarguments, then such a withdrawal becomes more problematic. When it comes to one's own career, preserving friendships or raising children, this kind of reticence is hardly an option in many cases. If even the health of loved ones is at stake, then objectivity and composure are usually a thing of the past anyway.

Discussion patterns of this kind, in which facts simply do not help, do not only occur, as in the case of poor Sophie, with the followers of conspiracy myths, pseudoscience and alternative medicine. Very similar situations can also be experienced with religious fundamentalists, the followers of sectarian communities, and even political extremists. So, such challenges are not new, and there are also quite a number of considerations on how to help oneself. From the philosophical perspective of logic, for example, the issue is how to separate scientific from unscientific thinking under everyday conditions [1] or how to avoid common logical fallacies [2]. From the more rhetorical side, there are instructions on how to break through typical argumentation patterns of believers on the basis of concepts such as street epistemology [3] or subversive thinking [4] and, if necessary, enter into a fruitful dialogue after all. The authors of such approaches are sometimes very optimistic about the chances of success of their ideas. However, all these concepts presuppose a minimum of cooperation and accessibility to logical arguments on the part of the other party, as well as an acknowledgement of a common factual basis.

In this book, we follow a very practical approach: we are guided by the experience of people who are or have been forced into such argumentations particularly often, including especially those who have once been on the other side themselves. From the transformation processes that people have gone through themselves, we can learn a lot about how to initiate or support such a challenging process in discussions and where the limits are. Based on this, we will take a closer look at some typical discussion situations and consider experiences in them as well as opportunities, objectives and limits of communication, and finally derive a few more or less generally applicable practical tips.

First of all, however, we will have to familiarize ourselves with some basic psychological effects that one can encounter again and again in discussions of this kind and for which one should be prepared in one's own argumentation and expectations.

References

1. Mukerji N (2016) Die 10 Gebote des gesunden Menschenverstands. Springer, Heidelberg
2. Richardson J et al (2020) Thou shalt not commit logical fallacies. https://yourlogicalfallacyis.com. Accessed on: 27. Jan. 2020
3. Boghossian PG (2013) A manual for creating atheists. Pitchstone, Durham
4. Schleichert H (2011) Wie man mit Fundamentalisten diskutiert, ohne den Verstand zu verlieren: Anleitung zum subversiven Denken, 7. Aufl. Beck, München

2

Why Do They Believe This? And Why Might We Believe Something Equally Nonsensical?

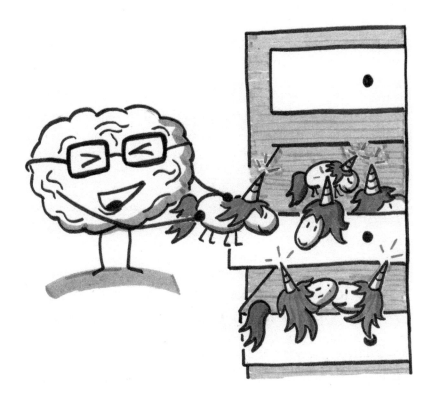

© The Author(s), under exclusive license to Springer-Verlag GmbH,
DE, part of Springer Nature 2022
H. G. Hümmler, U. Schiesser, *Fact and Prejudice*,
https://doi.org/10.1007/978-3-662-66032-4_2

In a Viennese coffee house I (Ulrike Schiesser) meet Krista Federspiel, who as a journalist, author and co-founder of the Austrian Skeptics Organization has had countless discussions with representatives of irrational world views. She tells me about the psi tests conducted by skeptic organizations worldwide. In these, people who claim to have a psychic ability can undergo scientific testing. If they pass all the test procedures, a prize money of €10,000 beckons at first and even a million dollars in the further course. If a paranormal force were to exist beyond doubt, it would revolutionize science and lead to countless research projects and applications – a fascinating thought and a potential source of income for scientists as well.

So diviners with pendulums, dowsers who claim to detect water veins, magnets or buried gold, fortune tellers and people who are convinced that they can read minds, heal or communicate with animals will apply. In the preliminary discussion the form of the examination is specified together; then the great day of the test comes, and in the consequence the sobering realization that the asserted abilities cannot withstand an examination with scientific standards. The candidates usually react at first with astonishment, irritation, shock. They honestly believed in these powers. Some are still stubbornly convinced of their effectiveness on the spot, others initially go home disillusioned. But the very next day the world looks quite different again. They find reasons why the test didn't work that particular day, explain that the skeptical attitude of the examiners was a negative influence, or that their ability fundamentally defies any verification. After only a few hours, almost all of them are again unswervingly convinced of the effectiveness of their psychic abilities. "You can't convince a true believer," is Krista Federspiel's sober conclusion.

Why is that? Why do people, even when directly confronted with evidence to the contrary, persist in their point of view? To answer this question, we need to look at how our perception, thinking and judgment work and are prone to error.

2.1 Emotions Determine Cognitive Processes, Affect Heuristics

We like to think of ourselves as logical beings, convinced of our abilities to perceive the world factually correct and to draw the right conclusions from it. Yet even our perception is highly subjective and prone to error, our thought processes are largely determined by factors that have nothing to do with logic, and our values and emotions play a much more significant role than we realize. In short, we feel first and think second. We often use our intellect afterwards to justify our previously formed opinion. Emotions determine our actions much more strongly than information.

In 2016, a group of American neuroscientists monitored the brain activity of subjects in a magnetic resonance imaging scanner while they were presented with information that conflicted with their political beliefs. Even during simpler challenges to their beliefs, areas of the brain typically involved in processing complex information were active, along with areas involved in social interaction. The stronger the attacks on political beliefs became, the more brain areas that otherwise become active primarily during fear and physical threat also stirred [1].

The strategists of the advertising industry have long since adapted to this and use these mechanisms professionally. When buying a car, the technical facts play a subordinate role compared to the "feel-good vibes" that the product must spread. Laughing, happy people, freedom, family, adventure, eroticism, the image of the brand in question … these are the promises that commercials convey to us; by contrast, fuel consumption, breakdown statistics and environmental compatibility take up hardly any space.

There is a content level and a relationship level in every communication. The relationship level is an important factor in the reception of information. The communication scientist Paul Watzlawick used the image of an iceberg: only 20% are visible, which corresponds to the factual level, the exchange of facts. But communication is strongly co-determined by the 80% underwater, the feelings, the relationships, the social and cultural influences. If there is a disturbance in the relationship, this also has a disturbing effect on the factual level (iceberg model). To reach people, it is not enough to address facts. You have to understand and address their emotions. What is behind the views they hold? What fears, concerns, motives? If these are not addressed, the information often does not reach its target.

Our society is based on trust to a much greater extent than we ourselves realize: Trust in the expertise of others, trust in science, trust in government institutions. The vast majority of all those facts that we call our knowledge cannot be verified by ourselves. Can water store information? Have humans landed on the moon? Is genetic engineering dangerous? Unless you are an expert in that field, you have to rely on what you hear about it from others. You have to trust that the textbooks convey correct facts, that the media report truthfully, that there is verified factual knowledge that comes from independent universities and research institutes and is expanded. Your worldview is largely shaped by which source of information you trust. We speak of the "perceived truth."

Conspiracy myths corrode this trust. They assume that there are large-scale conspiracies that permeate and corrupt all the main pillars of the state and society. Citizens would be deceived with systematic misinformation, while shady powers operate in the background. In this worldview, every fact, every statement and every piece of information appears dubious, even directly suspect. The film "The Matrix" by the Wachovskis from 1999 sums up this basic feeling most clearly. Everything that appears to us as reality is in truth a virtual projection to keep us docile and exploit us. The more such world views spread, the more difficult it becomes to reach people with information and education, and the easier it is for demagogues to play. In the worst case, the common consensus about our reality is lost.

2.2   Errors in Our Perception

Moonrise: The moon disk stands huge above the horizon. But the further it climbs up the night sky, the smaller it appears to us.

The sensory organs provide an enormous amount of data, which is condensed, categorized and interpreted in the brain. In this process, our perception is already influenced by our experiences and expectations. Over time, our brain develops processing routines that serve faster and more energy-efficient processing. We see the world not as it objectively is, but as we expect to find it based on our experience (see Fig. 2.1).

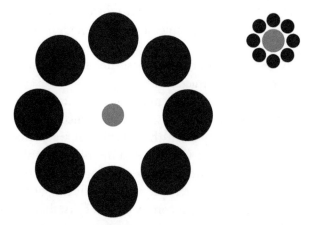

Fig. 2.1 A well-known example of the susceptibility of our perception to be deceived was developed by the psychologist Hermann Ebbinghaus: The two gray circles are the same size, even though they appear to us to be different sizes. (Own illustration based on the idea of Ebbinghaus)

The developmental psychologist Martin Doherty has shown in an experiment that children are less susceptible to these perceptual illusions than adults because their brains still have less experience stored to fall back on. It still has to analyze sensory impressions with more precision and effort. Adults see the world more imprecisely and with more errors than they did as children [2].

Pareidolia

Sometimes misinterpretations of the provided data arise, for example when a matching image is constructed from random elements: Figures can be recognized in clouds, the moon seems to have a face, even a spot on the wall can resemble a figure. Behind the technical term pareidolia is the ability of our brain to construct a meaningful figure from random elements. Faces are put together particularly frequently in this process (see Fig. 2.2). This may once have had evolutionary advantages, when the movement of leaves in the forest

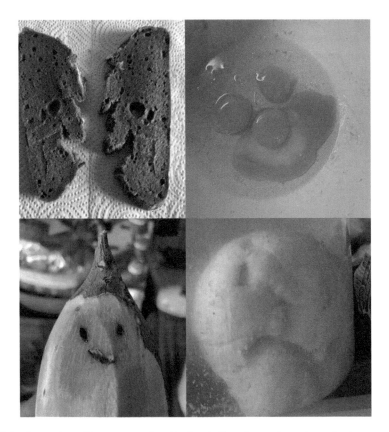

Fig. 2.2 Examples of faces recognized in foods (farmhouse bread, cracked eggs, sweet potato, mozzarella). (Photographs: Susanne Schiesser, Brigitte Michlmayr)

was quickly identified as a predator. In any case, it again shows the tendency of our brain to quickly sort impressions into appropriate categories and patterns, and even in chaotic structures, to search overzealously for order, for meaningful content.

Michael Shermer puts it this way, *"Our brains are belief engines: evolved pattern-recognition machines that connect the dots and create meaning out of the patterns that we think we see."* [3].

This can also be lucrative. In 2004, Diane Duyser of Florida auctioned off a slice of toast on which she claimed to recognize the face of St. Mary for $28,000, and as early as 1978, a tortilla in New Mexico purporting to have Jesus on it drew crowds of devotees.

However, pareidolia are not only entertaining, but clearly contribute to irrational belief systems. For example, former ghost hunter Hayley Stevens now explains a large portion of the circulating ghost photos, some of which she herself used to believe in, as pareidolia. In 1976, many people recognized a face in an image of the Martian surface sent by NASA's Viking-1 spacecraft. Twenty-five years later, a much more accurate image of the roughly 1.5-km-wide structure from the Mars Global Surveyor probe showed it to be simply a crumbling rock formation (see Fig. 2.3). Nevertheless, a conspiracy myth that circulates among right-wingers and esotericists to this day claims that NASA is covering up that the face is evidence of an extraterrestrial culture that also built the Egyptian and Mexican pyramids [4]. In 2012, UFO believers

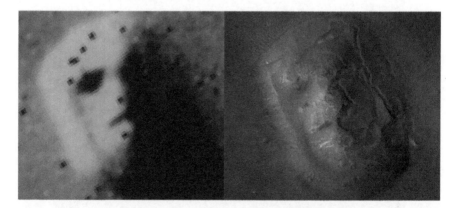

Fig. 2.3 The so-called face on Mars photographed by the 1976 Viking 1 (left) and 2001 Mars Global Surveyor (right). The impression of a face on the Viking image is due to shadows cast by flat incident sunlight and pixels lost in the data transfer and rendered in black. The Mars Global Surveyor image was taken at a much more favorable sun angle. (Image copyright: NASA)

thought they had spotted a rat or squirrel on a photograph taken by the Mars probe Curiosity [5].

Food for Thought

When you look at the images with the food or the Martian face, can you escape the impression of actually having faces in front of you? How would that impression change if you were in a supposedly haunted castle at night and recognized a similar face in wisps of fog, a torn curtain, or an old grandfather clock?

2.3 Error in Memory

My (Ulrike Schiesser's) sister Klara tells the story of being involved in a car accident when she was 16. The car skids on a curve in heavy snowfall, slides off the roadway and comes to a stop, with the front wheels already partially over a slope. The driver and front passenger get out immediately to reduce the weight in front, and the three backseat passengers remain seated to prevent the car from tipping forward while help is summoned. My sister sits in the back seat and describes the following 10 min as extremely stressful and anxiety-provoking. An impressive experience, an exciting story that she still tells years later. Until a friend interrupts her in astonishment: "Klara, you weren't even there!" My sister is irritated and perplexed. She remembers the situation so well, the fear and the relief when a tractor finally secured the vehicle. She is completely sure that she experienced it herself. But she didn't, as it turns out. She empathized with the stories told by the victims at the time, put herself in their shoes, and after a few years this empathic experience was mixed with real memories and stored as a biographical element. Without her being aware of it, a false memory has crept in.

Narratives like this abound. Our memory is not a static structure like a library in which individual elements are managed like book entries, but a dynamic process. We construct memories anew each time we recall them, and this is an error-prone process, even if we try hard to reproduce them correctly. In psychotherapy, self-awareness sessions, or trance experiences, repressed and forgotten memories can be brought back to consciousness, but they can also lead to false memories that are indistinguishable from real ones through manipulative conversation, staging, and the right choice of words (priming).

In police interviews, this effect becomes well visible, and great care must be taken not to influence the statements by asking certain questions. Emotionally stressful experiences are particularly susceptible to manipulation. In an experiment, the psychologist Julia Shaw succeeded in persuading people that they had committed a crime as teenagers. Using appropriate conversational techniques, the subjects were able to describe in detail and convincingly an event that never happened and were themselves convinced of its veracity [6].

2.4   Fast Thinking/Slow Thinking

Can you remember your first driving lesson? How highly concentrated you had to be at every gear change, how exhausting it was to keep an eye on the driving speed, the road, traffic signs and other road users at the same time and to react appropriately and correctly to the many stimuli. After a few years of driving experience, all this hardly costs you any energy anymore; you do it automatically without consciously thinking about it. You can even listen to an audio book or make a phone call or sing a song at the same time. But if you are looking for an address for the first time in left-hand traffic in London, you will switch off the audio book; if you are supposed to make a decision on a complex problem in a telephone call, you will park before continuing to speak; this also applies if you compose the song yourself.

According to the psychologist and Nobel Prize winner Daniel Kahneman, there are, roughly speaking, two variants of how our brain can solve thinking tasks [7]:

- **System 1:** fast, automated, emotional, pigeonholes, runs unconsciously, costs little energy. Examples are: driving a car (unless you are a novice driver); recognizing our favorite song; knowing that the church on the horizon is bigger than our hand, even though it looks smaller; recognizing an angry facial expression; continuing the words "In God we …". In order to effectively process the large amount of information we are confronted with every day, we form a category system. All it takes is a small detail of appearance, and immediately a person is pigeonholed into one of these categories. This happens automatically, is convenient, and is rarely questioned. This shortcut also makes perfect sense. Our complex everyday life would not be manageable if we wanted to examine every single piece of information we are confronted with as if we were hearing the fact for the very first time, realign our world view with every discussion, and act as if encountering a new species for the first time with every encounter with a person.
- **System 2:** must be consciously activated, works slowly, costs energy, is based on logic and conscious thought processes, but is not immune to mistakes. This system becomes active, for example, when we are solving a crossword puzzle, trying to match a face that seems familiar, choosing the new sofa for the living room, waiting for the traffic light to turn green,

picking the most beautiful apple from the bowl. These thinking tasks require much more energy and concentration; you cannot do several of these System 2 tasks in parallel. For example, you cannot formulate a text in parallel with solving a math problem. Whether you can carry on a conversation while knitting depends on whether you are a beginner and how complex the pattern is. If you are counting stitches, the conversation is on pause.

According to Kahneman, we tend to overestimate ourselves and make errors in thinking, but are under the illusion that we are acting competently, rationally, and logically. We prefer simple explanations to complex ones, are fundamentally lazy about thinking, and also like to take the path of least resistance when making judgments.

2.5   Cognitive Biases

On television, an expert discussion is taking place about the effectiveness of homeopathy. Opinions differ in the Wegner family. Mrs. Wegner is convinced of its efficacy; the globules have alleviated her persistent skin rash, improved her sleep, and dog Bello's arthritis has become much better. Her daughter Valerie is convinced that the successes of homeopathy are only placebo effects and considers the alleged mechanisms of action to be nonsense. In her medical studies, she became involved in an initiative that wants to remove homeopathy lectures at the university. Mr. Wegner is undecided; he can understand both sides. For months, his wife and daughter have been trying to convince the other of their own point of view. Internet links to relevant articles, sites and discussion forums are exchanged without success. Even after the TV discussion, both are sure that their own position has provided the far better arguments and convinced the viewers. Both see themselves confirmed in their opinion.

Confirmation bias describes the experience that only those facts are taken on board that strengthen one's own views; others are weakened or ignored. We hold on to our opinions more firmly, the more they are emotionally significant and part of a broader world view. This filtering sieve is already at work in perception, influencing how we interpret and store data and how we remember it. The confirmation bias becomes active especially when it comes to basic attitudes and values of a person and when the topic seems important to us. Changing one's position would lead to far-reaching shifts in our view of the world and our self-image. This costs energy, is often associated with feelings of shame, and is therefore largely avoided.

We insert new information into an already existing worldview, keeping it as constant as possible. This includes our political and religious attitudes, our value systems, our explanatory models, our basic experience of how the world affects us and how we can be effective in this world. This view of the environment is partly formed in childhood, may have been shaped by the attitudes of parents, or may have been formed in conscious opposition to them. Were parents more concerned with preserving the familiar and more fearful and suspicious of change, or did they enthusiastically embrace the new and strange, valuing diversity and innovation? Did they believe that everyone is the architect of his own fortune or that we are controlled by the powers "up there" and that fate, God or other external influences control our lives? Without realizing it, we adopt many basic attitudes from the first formative environment of our childhood and youth.

The culture in which we grow up, the social environment, but also the attitudes we develop in the course of our lives create the glasses through whose tint we look at the world. Everything we perceive is colored by this filter. In the process, our attitude seems so natural to us that we perceive it as THE reality, and we are usually not even aware that it is an interpretation of reality created by us. The confrontation with other world views is a valuable expansion of our perspectives. However, the first reactions that usually arise are irritation, defensiveness, and a posture to fight for our own worldview. We prefer to surround ourselves with people who share our worldviews. This confirms us, creates security and a sense of belonging. This is particularly visible in social media, which further reinforces the emergence of such social bubbles. It feels comfortable in our shared nest of beliefs. We know who the good guys and the bad guys are, we agree. Our attitudes are shared and constantly reinforced by others, and echo chambers are created, confronting us less and less with alternative views. If these views appear, then as a common enemy that is despised, to be fought against. Black-and-white thinking is reinforced; there is also the impression (or the concrete experience) of losing membership in one's own group as soon as one holds a dissenting opinion. For example, if you post a change of heart in the Facebook group of vaccination opponents, you are quickly expelled from the group. People prefer to keep to themselves and avoid the strenuous confrontation with other points of view. Too quickly, a dissenting opinion is experienced as a personal attack.

2.6   Judgment Heuristics: Pigeonhole Thinking

Heuristics describe a multitude of thinking routines how to form an opinion or find a solution as easily as possible either with little information or with an overabundance of information. They are, so to speak, a shortcut in the analysis process.

Psychologist Klaus Fiedler [8] describes them this way:

> Heuristics are cognitive tools that enable social individuals to make judgments through simplified "rules of thumb" that do not require a great deal of effort, but often lead to quite good results.

The unwieldy term **cum hoc ergo propter hoc** refers to the fallacy that if two things happen at the same time, there must be a cause-and-effect relationship: *"The number of storks is going down. The number of births is going down. This is evidence that storks are bringing babies."*

Tyler Vigen [9] collects and presents on his website a large number of these so-called spurious correlations (more correctly: spurious causalities), for example that the consumption of margarine in the USA is highly correlated with the divorce rate in the US state of Maine (r = 0.992; see Fig. 2.4). From this, a regional newspaper, let's call it "Daily Prophet Maine," could derive a

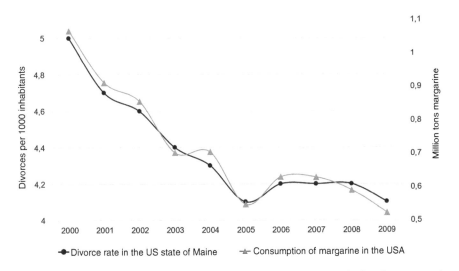

Fig. 2.4   The correlation of margarine consumption in the U.S. with the divorce rate in the state of Maine from 2000 to 2009. (Own graph based on US Census Bureau data, correlation detected by www.tylervigen.com)

tip for couples: *"The less margarine on the table, the longer your marriage will last. Butter makes for happy love!"*

The fallacy under the name **post hoc ergo propter hoc** is similar: because one event follows another, the first must be the cause of the second.

"After I took Arnica D30, the fever went down." The fever could have gone down all by itself because that is the usual course of the disease or because another medicine was taken. *"Just now I was thinking about my aunt, and she calls me! I must have anticipated this."* Not considered here is how often one thought of the aunt without her picking up the phone.

The more retrievable a piece of information is to our memory, the more easily we remember an event, the more likely and correct we judge it to be. This is where the **availability bias** comes into play. What is familiar seems to be true. The more frequently a particular memory content is accessed, the more pronounced the corresponding memory trace becomes. We create cognitive pathways in the brain. Imagine a summer meadow; if you cross it once, the grass soon straightens out, but if you tread the same path again and again, a trail slowly emerges, and over time, a distinct path. Automatically, you will now choose that path rather than trying to make another one through the grass.

We are more likely to remember things that we have readily available, that are often reported; for example, car accidents, violent crimes, and environmental disasters are considered more dangerous than heart attacks, diabetes, and strokes because these extraordinary incidents are reported more frequently in the media. In real terms, many more people die from health problems than from violent influences.

The less effort it takes to remind us of something, the more likely it seems to be true. Propaganda and advertising also work with repetition.

Even with misinformation and myths, frequent repetition can make the information seem more plausible to us. The clearly disproven claim that vaccination can cause autism is familiar to many people because of its frequent mention, and thus remains in the memory. The dilemma of those who want to counter false claims is that they make this false information more widely known simply by mentioning it, thereby increasing its impact. This is called the **Familiarity Backfire Effect.**

In 2012, when the widespread concern in esoteric circles arose that the end of the world was coming because the Mayan calendar would supposedly "end" on that day, a frequently mentioned argument from unsettled people was, *"Actually, I don't believe it, but there are already so many books about it now and so many reports in the media and on the Internet, there must be some truth to it."*

Where there is a lot of smoke, there must be a fire, is a well-known fallacy that is also often cited in conspiracy myths.

A characteristic of a person – that can be the appearance, a hobby, a certain feature – radiates on the overall impression. People who are overweight, for example, are seen as less intelligent and more lazy, while attractive people are seen as more competent, honest and assertive. One characteristic creates something like a "halo," hence the name **halo effect**, which outshines other characteristics. Advertising uses prominent people to sell a product. The image of the idol is supposed to transfer to the product. In medical diagnosis, factors such as gender, ethnicity, age, sexual orientation, weight, and socioeconomic status act as influencing factors on the diagnosis of diseases [10].

When something is presented attractively in a beautiful design, it seems more correct to us. Conversely, a spelling error in the text makes the entire content seem less believable. For the same content, better grades are given with nicer handwriting. Easy comprehensibility and good visual presentation of a text increase the illusion of truth. Especially as soon as a picture supports a statement, the statement appears more credible to us. Pictures help to absorb and store information. At the same time, they convey (apparent) evidence that something has actually taken place, actually exists.

Such judgment heuristics can have very real effects on people's lives. For example, in the early 2000s, only 14.5% of all American men were taller than 1.83 m (6 ft), but among top executives at the largest companies, 58% were [11]. A clear correlation between height and income can also be demonstrated for men and women in Germany [12]. In the case of women, it is also noticeable that slimmer women achieve a higher income on average [13]. This is especially true for positions where leadership skills are more important than technical qualifications. The effect also only occurs with employed managers, not with successful company founders such as Mark Zuckerberg (Facebook), Jeff Bezos (Amazon) or Sergey Brin (Google), who are all below average in height. So body size apparently has a halo effect on perceived leadership quality, where a substantive relationship would be hard to justify factually.

Food for Thought

Put together like this, judgment heuristics, "cognitive biases," and quick thinking seem like design flaws in our brains. But just think for a moment about the last half hour before you opened this book today. How many times have you assumed without any verification that your family is really your family, that the black liquid from your pot is coffee, or that the object that looked like your chair is actually sturdy enough to sit on?

How would you cope in your daily life if you never wanted to make rash assumptions?

2.7   Cognitive Dissonance

Sarah K. has spent €28,000 over the past four years training as a medium with healer YX. Every month she has made a weekend pilgrimage to the teacher, who lives 400 km away, has strictly adhered to the dietary instructions that would be necessary to strengthen her energy body, has carried out the numerous exercises at home and has already worked with her own clients using the healer's method. Increasingly, however, doubts now arise as to whether this decision was the right one. The promised successes have so far failed to materialize, and the person of the healer seems to her more and more unsympathetic and unserious. Was the training a mistake? All that money and effort for nothing? Sarah doesn't even want to think about that; she pushes the doubts aside, labels them as resistance of the "ego" against the spiritual path and throws herself into her training with even more enthusiasm.

Cognitive dissonance is the name given to this unpleasant feeling when we fear we have made a mistake, when doubts arise about a decision, when a previous commitment is called into question. It describes the inner state of tension that arises when our behavior is not consistent with our values, when an investment yields less profit than expected, an action is more arduous than anticipated, when a decision turns out to be wrong, when we are disappointed or frustrated about something we ourselves have chosen.

The resulting feelings of failure, shame, and regret are very uncomfortable. We feel stupid, pitiful, immoral. It causes stress to have possibly been wrong as well as wasted money and energy. And because this inner tension is hard to bear, we immediately do everything we can to reduce it. We start looking for arguments why a decision might have been good and right after all. We struggle to maintain a consistent self-image, wanting to be able to continue looking in the mirror. But since it is easier to change our thinking than our behavior, we tend to match our thoughts to our actions. Doubts are suppressed and often masked by particularly strong commitment to the cause. Information that justifies the previous attitude is preferred over critical information. What doesn't fit is made to fit; sometimes with a crowbar. Then unpleasant information is avoided, people who criticize are discredited, culprits are sought.

Dissonance can occur, for example,

- When our actions do not match our self-image,
- when a decision turns out to be wrong,
- when we receive negative information about a person, idea, action we value,

- when success fails to materialize, unexpected obstacles arise, or an expectation is not met.

This effect was first formulated by psychologist Leon Festinger. He had infiltrated a group led by Marian Keech, a Salt Lake City medium, in the 1950s. She was convinced that all of humanity would be destroyed by a massive flood and that only the members of her group would be saved by aliens in UFOs. Her followers had campaigned in advance, aggressively recruiting members, in some cases giving up all possessions, and investing a great deal of commitment and their personal reputations in this belief. Festinger joined these people in waiting for the end of the world and the spaceship on D-day. Midnight came and passed – no flood, no aliens. Festinger was curious to see how the group would react. How would they manage to face their skeptical relatives, media, and work colleagues the next day, from whom they had said goodbye forever the day before? To his astonishment, only some of the members turned away from the leader and the group; most of them intensified their commitment even more afterwards. The end of the world had not come, only because the community had prevented it with their prayers. This demonstrated the power and moral superiority of the group.

To reduce cognitive dissonance, people resort to the following methods:

- Suppressing: denying the importance of the topic.
- Devaluing the persons concerned: For example, a victim of violence is accused of having only himself or herself to blame, of being a second-class person.
- Upvaluing one's own behavior: I am a warrior of light, I do this for the good of all humanity. My behavior is significant, even if others cannot see it. The doubters are not yet "awakened", do not have a higher consciousness.

People who were members of cult-like groups often report that after the first doubts about the infallibility of the guru were awakened, they became particularly intensely committed to the community. They experienced these doubts as threatening, as a personal flaw, or as the input of an outside evil force, and they responded with increased commitment to the community.

2.8   Anecdotal Evidence

Franziska R. was diagnosed with pancreatic cancer. The doctor at the hospital advised her to get her affairs in order; in five years, she could only expect a 10% chance of survival. Desperate, she seeks help from Karl F., who works with quantum healing. "Forget about these numbers," he tells her, "only yesterday I had an elementary school teacher, 45 years old, mother of two children, who was already given up by the doctors! She was given only a few weeks to live. Then I started to treat her. After half a year the metastases were reduced by half, and after five years she was declared cured. And she is not the only one. I experience miracles like this all the time. When should I start treatment?"

A story that we can identify with and that triggers emotions in us is more convincing than statistics. If it also promises us an outcome we desire, this narrative unfolds especially great power. Like the story of Markus, a carpenter's apprentice, who became rich thanks to the online marketing tool of success coach XY, or the report of Anna, who lost 12 kg in three weeks with the help of a miracle berry, or the comment on the homepage by Mrs. Wieser, who finally has the strength to live again thanks to the services of the witch Walpurga, because she has removed an evil curse from her. No matter in which area, the use of personal narratives touches us especially deeply. We identify with these people, rejoice with them, and fill up with hope that we too could succeed in what is so enthusiastically described there.

If you want to reach people, you have to tell them a good story. This is also known as the "person who" fallacy. "I know someone who ....", "Smoking can't be that unhealthy, my grandpa lived to be 92 and smoked like a chimney his whole life."

Aside from the fact that case stories are often fabricated, individual cases are never informative of statistical probabilities. But people generally have a hard time with these probabilities. We are very bad at realistically assessing dangers, fearing air travel more than car travel, for example, even though the numbers clearly show that there is a higher risk of dying in a car accident. Cows cause more deaths worldwide than sharks: the alpine pasture nevertheless seems to us a much safer place than the sea.

Would you have known? About 10 people die each year from shark attacks, around 150 from jellyfish, an estimated 25,000 from dogs, 100,000 from snakes, 725,000 from mosquitoes that carry diseases like malaria [14].

2.9   Peer Pressure

Imagine you are sitting in a room with several other people; three lines of different lengths are projected on the wall, with another next to it for comparison. Your task is to select that line that is the same length as the reference line. It is a simple task. The lines clearly have different lengths, and you find the right one right away, number two. Before you are asked, the other participants in the study (who are actually co-workers of the study director) state their result. Everyone agrees that it is line number three. How will you answer? Only a quarter of the subjects never change their minds in favor of the group opinion; the majority forgo their own perceptions and go along with the majority. The larger the group, the more likely you are to adjust your opinion. However, if even one more person decides against the group opinion and chooses a different solution, the subject's courage to insist on his own perception also increases.

This experiment was first conducted by psychologist Solomon Asch in 1951 and has been repeatedly confirmed since then [15]. We are influenced by the judgments, values, and attitudes of our environment. In groups, we tend to go along with the prevailing opinion and behave in conformity. This effect is particularly effective when it is a group we identify with, want to be recognized by, or depend on. Behind this is the desire to be accepted and not excluded. In one's own place of residence, especially a village, all three factors are at work: one does not want to attract negative attention, does not want to strain relations with neighbors, and, out of solidarity with friends, also supports positions that one might not otherwise hold. The stronger the longing for recognition and belonging, the greater the willingness to adopt the norms and opinions of a group. The willingness to adopt group norms also increases in the face of stress and threat, as well as in the face of a lack of information.

Of course, as part of a group, we are not only influenced by the group – we are, after all, part of the group at the same time and allow our ideas and values to flow into the group norms. But the group is not simply the sum of its members, and, contrary to what is often thought, not only in a positive sense. Experiments have shown time and again that, in the case of objectively measurable performance of an equal type, groups perform significantly worse than the sum of their individual members. At the same time, through division of labor and the use of different skills, groups can accomplish feats that the members would not be able to do individually. In a tug-of-war, groups tend to perform worse than their individual members; but building a house is only possible when people work together, some of whom can build walls and others can lay water pipes or cables.

But groups also think differently than single individuals. In groups, people tend to support and encourage each other. As a result, people more easily tune out concerns – both concerns about the risks they are taking and moral reservations. This phenomenon, called **groupthink**, is often exemplified by political decisions made in cabinets or advisory councils. Popular examples include the failed invasion of Cuba by exiled Cuban rebels with the support of the U.S. government under President Kennedy, the failure to defend Pearl Harbor before U.S. entry into World War II, or the assumption that Iraq still had weapons of mass destruction at the start of the second Gulf War. It is striking, however, that other possible explanations are put forward for all three examples and that the assessment depends strongly on one's own political attitude. The phenomenon itself has also been confirmed in psychological experiments, however, and it could also lead, for example, to the fact that people who all on their own have only a slight tendency to believe in conspiracies can nevertheless become strongly radicalized in a group. Groups whose members are very similar to each other and who are relatively closed off to the outside world seem to be particularly susceptible to groupthink [16]. As will also become apparent when looking at successful transformation processes, followers of alternative medicine and conspiracy myths in particular tend very strongly to separate themselves from supposedly ignorant or even malicious outsiders. In turn, in such communities, a high degree of similarity among each other often results simply from the fact that we trust people more easily who are similar to us, for example, who have the same profession, the same hobbies or the same attitudes.

2.10 Social Framework

Of course, we are influenced not only by our individual thinking and by the group we are in at any given moment, but also by the environment and framework we live with, and also by those we have grown up with. Relatively obvious influences are education and social class – but it certainly also plays a role in the question of whether one expects healing more from nature or from science, whether one grew up in a more urban or more rural environment and what ideas have accordingly been conveyed not only by parents but also by neighborhood, teaching staff and circle of friends.

These influences have recently been researched, especially in connection with young people who join right-wing extremist or jihadist groups. It is apparent that such radicalization processes cannot, of course, be viewed separate from the social environment and tend to occur more frequently in an environment that is considered to be unfavorable. However, corresponding authors also point out that the same circumstances and the same political education regularly produce both democrats and radicals – and that a not inconsiderable proportion of right-wing extremist young people in particular come from the so-called "middle of society" [17].

These findings can certainly be applied in part to conspiracy thinking and other anti-scientific belief systems. The interrelationships here are often too complex and too little researched in detail to be summarized here. Simple, generalized statements like "East Germans believe more in conspiracies" are usually not confirmed in careful investigations [18]. However, one should always be clear: When you discuss with a person his or her rejection of science, you are always also fighting against influences that are outside of that person and possibly already far in the past.

> **Takeaway**
>
> As strange as esotericism, conspiracy beliefs, and religious or political fanaticism may seem to us, there are largely psychological mechanisms behind them that operate in each of us. These mechanisms are to a large extent useful for our everyday life, and to some extent even necessary for our survival. But they can also lead us up the garden path, justify and stabilize anti-scientific belief systems.
>
> And we fight against all these psychological mechanisms when we try to convince believers.

References

1. Kaplan JT et al (2016) Neural correlates of maintaining one's political beliefs in the face of counterevidence. Sci Rep 6:39589
2. Doherty M, Campbell N, Tsuji H, Phillips W (2010) The Ebbinghaus illusion deceives adults but not young children. In: Developmental science. Blackwell, Oxford, S 714–721. https://www.readcube.com/articles/10.1111%2Fj.1467-7687.2009.00931.x?purchase_referrer=onlinelibrary.wiley.com&tracking_action=preview_click&r3_referer=wol&show_checkout=1. Accessed on: 6. März 2021
3. Shermer M (2011) The believing brain: from spiritual faiths to political convictions – how we construct beliefs and reinforce them as truths. Robinson, London
4. Light A (2012) The 10th sumerian tablet: the Anunnaki built the pyramids. https://humansarefree.com/2012/12/the-10th-sumerian-tablet-the-anunnaki-built-the-pyramids.html. Accessed on: 12. Febr. 2021
5. Smith A (2013) Was a squirrel discovered on Mars? https://www.zdnet.com/pictures/was-a-squirrel-discovered-on-mars/. Accessed on: 12. Febr. 2021

6. Shaw J (2018) Das trügerische Gedächtnis: Wie unser Gehirn Erinnerungen fälscht. Heyne, München

7. Kahnemann D (2012) Schnelles Denken, langsames Denken. Siedler, München

8. Fiedler K (2014) Die Verarbeitung sozialer Informationen für Urteilsbildung und Entscheidungen. In: Jonas K, Stroebe W, Hewstone H (eds) Sozialpsychologie. Springer, Heidelberg, pp 143–175

9. Tyler Vigen: Spurious correlations (2021). https://www.tylervigen.com/spurious-correlations. Accessed on: 6. März 2021

10. Croskerry P, Nimmo GR (2011) Better clinical decision making and reducing diagnostic error. Review at the RCPE Patient Safety Hot Topic Symposium

11. Gladwell M (2005) Blink! – die Macht des Moments. Campus, Frankfurt a.M

12. Spanhel F (2010) Der Einfluss der Körpergröße auf Lohnhöhe und Berufswahl: Aktueller Forschungsstand und neue Ergebnisse auf Basis des Mikrozensus. Statistisches Bundesamt, Wiesbaden

13. Caliendo M, Gehrsitz M (2014) Obesity and the labor market: a fresh look at the weight penalty. Forschungsinstitut zur Zukunft der Arbeit, Berlin

14. Welt Wissen: Das sind die Topkiller unter den Tieren (2021). https://www.welt.de/wissenschaft/gallery131831471/Das-sind-die-Topkiller-unter-den-Tieren.html. Accessed on: 6. März 2021

15. Hewstone M, Martin R (2014) Sozialer Einfluß. In: Jonas K, Stroebe W, Hewstone H (eds) Sozialpsychologie. Springer, Heidelberg, pp 269–313

16. Park JW (1990) A review of research on groupthink. J Behav Decis Mak 3:229–245

17. Kleeberg-Niepage A (2012) Zur Entstehung von Rechtsextremismus im Jugendalter – oder: Lässt sich richtiges politisches Denken lernen? J Psychol 20(2):1–30

18. Bartoschek S (2017) Bekanntheit von und Zustimmung zu Verschwörungstheorien – eine empirische Grundlagenarbeit. jmb, Hannover

3

Transformation Processes

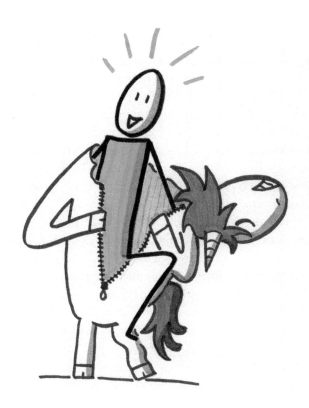

H. G. Hümmler, U. Schiesser, *Fact and Prejudice*,
https://doi.org/10.1007/978-3-662-66032-4_3

If you take on all these psychological effects when encountering a follower of an unscientific belief system, you should first ask yourself what you want to achieve. The obvious goal in such a discussion should actually be to convince one's opponent. The believer would have to give up his belief system, at least in single aspects, and be convinced by scientific evidence.

Those who think scientifically themselves will possibly find this a quite natural step. Doesn't one simply have to understand the methodology of scientific work and acquire the knowledge of research results or have them imparted to one? In the last section, however, it has already been shown what psychological obstacles stand in the way of such a transformation of beliefs. In addition, science is often not understood by believers as the method of critical thinking, constant questioning and mutual control that it is or at least should be. Whereas scientists usually take it for granted that scientific knowledge will only hold until it is replaced by better knowledge, believers often have a fundamentally different view of science: scientific knowledge is perceived as beliefs to be learned from textbooks and not to be doubted [1]. As a consequence, one's own beliefs are classified as at least equivalent, if not superior, because they are supported by personal experience. Nevertheless, even abstruse belief systems such as clairvoyance and spiritual healing strive for recognition by science, while at the same time rejecting it as a means of achieving knowledge [2]. To reconcile both, often adventurous distortions of scientific theories, for example of quantum mechanics or systems theory, have to be used, which are presented as the latest state of research [3]. Thus, believers often do not see themselves as opponents of science at all, but rather as ahead of the current, purely materialistic state of research.

After all, even otherwise scientifically skeptical people always manage to create mental niches for scientifically untenable doctrines, especially if these are easier to reconcile with their own values and ideologies than the actual state of science. In recent times, for example, there have been repeated clashes within the skeptic movement with climate change deniers or with people who completely deny social influences on gender roles. The conversely unscientific position of denying biological influences on gender roles, on the other hand, is unsurprisingly rarely encountered in the skeptic scene with its base in the natural sciences.

There are certainly current psychological studies on the short-term effects of individual discussions, educational campaigns, and similar interventions, and there are also repeated recommendations based on these (e.g., [4, 5]). Such interventions and effects can also be studied comparatively easily under controlled conditions. Fundamental transformation processes of beliefs towards a more scientifically based long-term view of the world, on the other hand, are a much more difficult object of research. In order to nevertheless be able to make statements about such processes, we have interviewed a number of people who have themselves experienced such a transformation. All of them once followed scientifically untenable convictions, some only in the context of a personal interest, while others earned their living with it. Some have become skeptical activists afterwards; others have only changed their personal behavior, but for all of them giving up their beliefs was a mental achievement for which different influencing factors played a role. We will trace these influences in this and the following sections and always try to learn from them.

3.1   From "Alternative Medicine" to Medicine

A Book Turns Out Quite Differently Than Expected

Probably the most prominent transformation process towards a scientific worldview in the recent past in Germany has been undergone by the physician **Natalie Grams**. As a physician with an official degree in homeopathy, she opened a homeopathic private practice in 2011. Around that time, she was interviewed by journalist Nicole Heißmann for a book on homeopathy. When the book was finally published under the title "The Homeopathy Lie," she was disappointed and wrote a negative review on Amazon. In the ensuing comment battle, she found herself confronted for the first time with the demand to prove that her perceived treatment successes were indeed a result of her homeopathic therapy. *"I never asked myself these questions before, and it was really such an aha moment, but not a pleasant one."* That's how she got the idea to write her own book: *"I felt like if there is this homeopathy lie, then someone has to write the homeopathy truth."* As, during the research for her own book, her doubts about beliefs long deemed certain grew, she sought clarity by contacting prominent homeopathy critics directly. To her amazement, those approached proved not only eager to provide information, but were also helpful and understanding. The book became a turning point in Natalie Grams' life, leading her to the forefront of a new movement of homeopathy critics, to the closure of her practice, and thus economically to a highly uncertain future. Discussions with skeptics on changing communication channels were thus not only the impetus for her transformation process that would last years, but played a central role over its entire period. With this, however, Natalie Grams is rather an exception, as will become apparent in the following.

At Some Point it Became Too Strange

The pediatrician **Thomas F.** was also a convinced follower of homeopathy during medical school. Introduced to it by fellow students, he was active in the homeopathy working group at his university, spent considerable sums on reference books and paid seminars on the subject, and tried to treat himself and his family with homeopathic globules: *"I really dived into it and was really in this bubble. There was no need at all to somehow take the outside perspective, because you felt comfortable and got along well with the people."* During this time, critical discussions happened only with his significant other, who was not from the medical field – and they came especially after he had unsuccessfully tried out his homeopathic healing skills on the child they had together. He always blamed his own mistakes for his continuing failure with homeopathy in his personal environment: Experienced, successful homeopaths, unlike him, could refer to a multitude of healing stories. The first impetus to break away from homeopathy finally came from the behavior of a fellow member of his own bubble, who began to get enthusiastic about Bach flower therapy: *"From the first moment I found that totally wacky and spooky."* The final turning point then came with the start of his professional career, when he perceived with alienation how an experienced colleague slipped into the world of "alternative medicine", did not vaccinate his children and finally opened a homeopathic practice. All in all, Thomas F.'s transformation process also took several years. Discussions of the kind we are interested in hardly played a role for him, because he almost never had them, but only lived out his faith among believers and in his family.

Driven to Research in Comment Battles

"I have advocated all kinds of garbage over the years, including homeopathy," explains **Florian Albrecht**, a physician. Above all, from today's perspective, mistletoe therapy for cancer, which originates from anthroposophical teachings, weighs heavily on him. Encouraged by a senior physician at his former clinic and by professional development courses, he recommended it to his patients. Today he fears that his recommendation may have massively worsened the outcome of treatment for at least two cancer patients who died shortly after mistletoe treatment despite originally having a good prognosis. While now he sometimes faces harsh criticism from other physicians because he insists on science-based treatments, his adventures in pseudo-medicine at that time only once met with opposition from colleagues or superiors: when

he wanted his clinic to pay the participation fee for a congress on psychedelic research, at which workshops on the "third eye" and on aura perception were offered, his head of department not only refused, but also canceled his already approved educational leave. However, the head of department himself liked to prescribe a specific type of homeopathy, and controversial procedures such as the Feldenkrais method were also used at the clinic. The trigger for Florian Albrecht's transformation was, of all things, a discussion with an anti-vaxxer: after a patient confronted him with hair-raising claims about adverse events from vaccination, he began to do research and came across skeptical and scientific online resources, especially on the portal Scienceblogs. Still in the role of a believer, he participated in the commentary discussions there and sometimes felt harshly attacked by scientifically skeptical discussion participants. When researching arguments for his ideas, he encountered mostly contradictory information when looking at reputable sources. As a result, he explains, he threw one alternative medical idea after another overboard in a daily or weekly rhythm. He now makes a point of no longer recommending or even prescribing unscientific therapies in his practice, and sees even parts of the skeptic scene as half-hearted and inconsistent when it comes to alternative medicine. In his case, then, discussions with skeptics have taken up some space, with his own research playing the decisive role in his relatively rapid transformation.

Why Is What I Do Forbidden?

Britt Marie Hermes is not a medical doctor, but completed a four-year college education in the USA as a naturopath, which, despite the much more extensive training, is roughly equivalent to a German *Heilpraktiker* in terms of the range of activities. She was then employed for several years in a naturopathic practice specializing in cancer patients, where patients were treated for a wide variety of tumors with the unapproved alleged miracle drug Ukrain. She deliberately avoided discussions with critics during this time. *"I didn't want to allow anything to infiltrate my mind."* She said she was convinced she was doing the right thing and that pharmaceutical companies were evil and doctors were untrustworthy. She says today that she knew surprisingly little about the drug she was predominantly using. She was all the more horrified when she discovered through an Internet search that it had no approval from drug regulators and that using such a drug on patients could be a crime under U.S. federal law. The fear of criminal prosecution prompted her to do more in-depth research, including coming across a book by critical complementary medicine professor Edzard Ernst, and eventually distancing herself from alternative medicine in direct exchanges with Ernst and other skeptical authors that lasted several months. As an important step she mentions the spatial separation from her previous environment, which had consisted almost exclusively of believers. Later, she became a skeptical activist, earned a doctorate in evolutionary biology, processed her experiences in a blog, and thus became the target of an unsuccessful libel suit by an American cancer healer [6]. So conversations with skeptics were very important to her transformation process, which she estimates to have taken about 9 months in total – but she didn't seek out these conversations until she was already well into her turnaround.

Never Really Felt Comfortable

You don't have to belong to a healing profession to take responsibility for someone else's health and get caught up in pseudoscientific ideas. Having become a mother at a very young age, **Theresa Stange** considered herself particularly skeptical when she insisted on having understood the meaning, effects and risks of vaccinations before having her baby vaccinated. However, she experienced the way her pediatrician at the time responded to what she now describes as mere insecurity not as reassuring, but as intimidating and reproachful. *"Then it was clear to me, okay, all this can't be right."* Searching for information on the Internet, she ended up primarily in anti-vaccination groups and, although she recognized some of the claims spread there as contradictory and naïve, they were enough to make doing nothing seem like the safer option. The children's father was an anti-vaccinationist on principle, with no real interest in further information, while she continued to research the Internet and buy books, but invariably ended up with sources from anti-vaccinationists. Thus, for years, not only the first but also the following child remained unvaccinated, and her own vaccination certificate also ended up in the waste paper. Nevertheless, Theresa Stange remained uneasy about her decision: she hardly dared to talk to other parents about the topic because she feared that her children might not be invited to birthdays or otherwise ostracized. She was happy whenever she met parents with children who were also unvaccinated. At the same time, she herself was aware that only talking to other parents about vaccinations which had gone normally, could have eased her fear. Even with her own sister, who has children of the same age, there were conflicts. The anti-vaccination group also provided only limited support: *"The people who wrote there, I thought to myself after a while, they're all not the* *brightest candles on the cake."* At the same time, medical advice that she recognized as irresponsible appeared regularly in the group, and critics were kicked out. A real change in thinking was only possible after she separated from the father of her children. Her new partner was an active skeptic and offered to obtain any information she wanted, including scientific evidence from experts if necessary, but otherwise deliberately held back and appeared to be a neutral authority, especially with regard to the children. Gradually, her feigned self-assurance gave way to more and more questions, to which she received well-founded answers. After a year, she first had her own vaccinations refreshed as a test and then had the children vaccinated as well. In her case, conversations with her new, well-informed life partner did indeed play an important role in the transformation process, but the uncertainty about her vaccine-critical attitude had been there before, actually always had; and yet the transformation took time.

3.2   Getting Out of the Conspiracy Swamp

Put off by the Scene

That even one's own partner is not always able to reach someone who is stuck in an unscientific belief system is shown by the example of **Stephanie Wittschier**. Fascinated by mysteries since her youth, the young woman saw a documentary on television about alleged inconsistencies surrounding the events of September 11. Curious, she began researching on the Internet and fell into what she calls a *"dangerous conspiracy swamp."* Soon she was believing not only in September 11 conspiracy myths, but also in chemtrails, mind control, right-wing anti-statist *"Reichsbürger"* ideology, a secret world government of alien reptilians and a hollow Earth inhabited by escaped Nazis. *"By the end, I really believed in almost everything, except the flat earth!"* [7] Criticism from her parents only led to her avoiding the subject to them. During this time, her husband repeatedly tried to point out to her the irrationality of her thinking. *"But I also just didn't listen to him at the time, and then I just showed him YouTube videos."* The first impetus to question her ideas came after 3 years, when a close friend from the scene turned away from conspiracy belief. But the decisive factor was ultimately the behavior in the scene itself: In a group of chemtrail believers, there was serious discussion about bringing down commercial airliners with laser pointers. When Stephanie Wittschier expressed her horror, she was thrown out of the group. She was expelled from another group after she supported a proposal for an experiment to look for chemical traces of chemtrails. The other chemtrail believers were not interested in serious testing of their claims. So Stephanie Wittschier began to question first her belief in chemtrails and then in the many other conspiracies. By now, she and her husband have initiated the page "The Loose Screw" and the group "Nothing but the Truth" on Facebook, where conspiracy myths are debunked, but also made fun of. She has strong words about her social environment at the time: *"These are not harmless weirdos. There are more areas in the conspiracy scene that are just as dangerous as the Reichsbürger scene, because everything merges."* So in Stephanie Wittschier's case, while she was still a believer, meaningful discussions were not possible at all – not even with her own husband.

For another conspiracy believer with a fairly similar history, who had also been deaf to her family, who had tolerated anti-Semitic diatribes and, even from her own point of view, absurd esoteric products at events, a photo became the impetus for her transformation. On the fact-checking portal mimikama.at, she discovered a picture that was frequently circulated in the scene, supposedly documenting the spraying of chemtrails. At Mimikama, she found proof that it was simply a fake. And even her first hand experience in the scene is of limited help when confronted with a conspiracy believer in her own family.

Converted by His Own Scientific Curiosity

Sebastian Bartoschek, a psychologist who wrote his doctoral thesis on conspiracy belief, often speaks sympathetically about believers, but online he is regarded as an equally provocative and astute campaigner, especially against political conspiracy thinking. He came to the topic, as he reports, as a believer himself. His youth was influenced by the ancient astronauts idea, i.e. Erich von Däniken's claims that extraterrestrial visitors in early human history were the basis for concepts of God, and he also picked up myths about the Holy Grail and conspiracy stories about the Kennedy assassination. Back then, before the boom of social media, he had many discussions, but he was not open to being convinced otherwise: *"It is a more comprehensive system than an individual belief. I found it particularly difficult to give up ancient astronauts, because that had become a part of my identity."* A change in thinking came about only during his studies and in the scientific examination of the subject. What he found helpful was the view of his later doctoral advisor that as a skeptic, one must also be able to admit if one has no explanation for an observation, but that that is also no proof for an arbitrary paranormal explanation.

The final turning away from ancient astronauts came during a trip to Mexico, when he stood in front of a Mayan fresco, on which, according to Däniken, an early historical astronaut should be seen. *"When I saw that then, in which overall context that stood and that he had picked out one of thousands of pictures, quite randomly, I had already been a sketical organization member for a long time, but then it finally clicked with me."* All in all, his transformation was a very gradual process that took almost 10 years. In the process, he increasingly interacted with skeptics and even became part of their movement before he was able to finally break away from his beliefs.

3.3   Losing My Religion

Why Don't Friends Tolerate It?

Another unnamed skeptic, who is still involved in the skeptical organization GWUP, even reports that only after years of activity in the skeptic movement he was ready to apply skeptical standards also to his own faith, in this case the Christian faith. Having grown up as a Catholic, for a long time he also considered apparitions of the Virgin Mary to be possible, for example. In the skeptic movement, he advocated exempting religious beliefs from skeptical scientific consideration. This exemption was the subject of fierce controversy at the time, and the skeptic found himself repeatedly under harsh personal attack, especially in e-mail discussions. *"That took a long time, but it did make a certain impression on me. I thought, they are actually quite nice and represent largely the same positions as I do. But why can't we agree on this issue? Why won't they tolerate it?"* Decisive for his turning away from faith had been personal experiences and the insight into the simple impossibility of what he believed in the context of the laws of nature, but these discussions had certainly also contributed to it. The disputes dragged on for several years, but the actual transformation finally took place within a few months, and precisely in a phase of such fierce controversies. So in his case, discussions actually made some contribution, but they were anything but sober and sympathetic.

The Others Are Happy Too

Lisa L. also comes from a religious family, but a much more restrictive one: She grew up with Jehovah's Witnesses. To please her parents, she was baptized at the – for the Witnesses' purposes – very young age of eight. At 15, she expressed doubts for the first time, which led not only to a severe crisis with her parents, but also to one-on-one study with an "elder" of the group. *"I had noticed time and time again that actually other people are happy, too."* Meanwhile, doubts grew silently, especially because of positions taken by Jehovah's Witnesses themselves, for example, about homosexuality: *"I didn't even have to say anything about it because they just presented it as fact, only I didn't take it as fact."* She was also put off by the Witnesses' hostility to education, including her mother who, despite having been to college, accepted the word of the Bible as the only truth. Important for her later detachment was the contact with outsiders, especially at school. There she not only had the opportunity to build friendships, but also to learn about and question new worldviews – a competence that was not welcome in Lisa's congregation. Above all, the ideals of the Enlightenment gave Lisa food for thought: *"Have the courage to use your own mind."* Finally, her two unbaptized older sisters, who had already completely renounced the faith before her, became key figures. The decisive factor here was *"that they accepted me as I am and not as I should be. I never had that feeling with Jehovah's Witnesses."* Her transformation process eventually lasted into young adulthood. Critical discussions about beliefs did not play a decisive role. Rather, what mattered was that outsiders were models for openness, tolerance, education, and personal happiness to her.

The Fear of One's Own Sainthood

Canadian **Jessica Schab** was not a follower of a religious cult – she was the cult. Feeling guilty about her father, who had claimed to be able to communicate with extraterrestrials and the deceased, after his death she also began to engage in contacts with the other side. After her first own videos, she was featured by a popular online channel and quickly gained an extensive following as "Jessicamystic" and "Crystal Child." At times, the YouTube channel with her messages about spirituality, aliens, the hollow earth and the machinations of the Illuminati had more than a million subscribers. She would not have been open to critical discussions during that time: *"For me, that was everything. It was my whole life! It was my livelihood! The amount of loss you have to endure in order to question is scary."* The trigger for her transformation, which she calls "unbrainwashing," eventually became confronting her own responsibility for her followers. During a conference in Spain, she was so irritated by the adoration she was receiving that she suddenly burped loudly as a spontaneous provocation. It was so inconceivable to bystanders that the crystal child could behave so rudely in public that they blamed her interpreter instead. *"That blew me away, but it wasn't enough to get me to question fully."* The time before the expected end of the world in 2012 she spent in Bali with crowds of other esoteric believers. In the process, she recognized many of the other spiritual leaders there as narcissists, cynics and profiteers – and many of her own followers as regular psychiatric patients. *"I wouldn't be able to live with myself, how would I have gone to bed at night, if I continued in that direction."* Only later in the course of her transformation over the coming years, critical conversations were able to help her find an identity for her to exist at all, independent of her faith. In addition to her partner at the time, who was a rationalist philosopher, help came from a documentary filmmaker who accompanied her journey over the years for the film "Confessions of a Former Guru". However, she has not completely let go of her former life to this day: *"There are times when it seems more appealing and easier just to go back to that. But I can't."* In all, it took her about 5 years to be able to detach herself from her faith at least that far. Critical conversations contributed to this only at relatively late stages, after it had already become clear to her that change was inevitable.

3.4   The Futile Search for the Paranormal

New Answers to Old Questions

A leading role in the esoteric scene, albeit on a much smaller scale, was also played by young Brit **Hayley Stevens**. Even as a teenager, she was fascinated by ghost sightings, as well as reports of monsters, psychics, and other paranormal phenomena. In her later teens, rather than relying solely on books and television reports, she formed her own ghost hunting team to search for spirits in alleged haunted houses with the consent of their respective owners. *"Looking back now, the whole thing was very biased, but at the time we weren't really aware of the logical mistakes that we were making."* Then, at about age 20, she realized there were other explanations for the observations that not only made more sense, but were more interesting than the same old methods of ghost hunting. *"I don't think it was just a complete change. I think that I was probably curious about these things, and becoming a ghost hunter was just how I happened to reach my conclusions."* What helped were discussions on Internet forums where skeptics were interested in the same phenomena, but in the process proposed their own, scientific explanations for them on an equal footing. For example, an unknown forum participant explained to her a supposed ghost photo with the pareidolia effect described in Sect. 2.2. *"I can remember getting really* *excited looking at the photographs we had taken as ghosthunters and going, oh my gosh, could this be the pareidolia effect?"* These clues became the starting point for her own research, which led her to new findings that were even more fascinating to her. Around the same time, one of her friends founded a skeptical podcast that introduced her to skeptical thinking and scientific ways of working. With her change in thinking, her ghost hunting team broke up under intense personal hostility between the group that wanted to do investigations according to scientific principles, and another, which continued to use Ouija boards,[1] spiritualist sessions and crystal pendulums. Within a year she had already begun to promote skeptical thinking as a blogger, podcaster and in lectures, in a form of engagement with her former environment that she herself sees as pejorative and cynical from today's perspective. Nowadays, she explains this to herself by her bitterness back then about the years and money she wasted as a ghost hunter. *"But that was my fault; that was nobody else's fault."* Now, studying psychology, she makes a point of addressing ghost believers on her blog, offering explanations rather than refuting claims. So discussions with skeptics were important for her rather quick transformations process from the very beginning – but that was possible mainly because in these discussions she found precisely the answers she had previously sought in vain as a ghost hunter.

A Single Book as an Eye Opener

That one can go through a rather similar process of changing one's mind even after achieving a certain academic status can be seen in the example of London psychology professor **Chris French**. In his youth, he was also fascinated by paranormal phenomena and at the time encountered only texts that presented such phenomena as facts. As a Ph.D. student, he made some money giving lectures in adult education, reporting, among other things, completely uncritically about supposedly sound results from parapsychology. Apart from that, however, he now remembers himself as a "silent believer" who hardly talked about it and therefore never got into discussions with skeptics. There still was no well-organized, publically active skeptics' movement at the time. Whenever in the media he got background information that for example the spectacular show effects presented by Uri Geller could be reproduced with common illusionist tricks, he found that irrelevant, simply because he was convinced that Geller wasn't using tricks. *"I just didn't see the relevance. Thinking about it*

---

[1] A Ouija board is a tablet with numbers and letters on which one tries to receive messages from the other world using a pointer guided by one or more persons with their hands.

today, I ask myself, how could I not see the relevance, but… that was it.” Then he encountered the book "Parapsychology - Science or Magic?" by Canadian psychologist James Alcock, which shows the fallacies and statistical weaknesses of that field of research. *"In Jim Alcock, I found the first consistent, well founded voice of skepticism and… it worked.”* French was convinced by the stringency of Alcock's scientific arguments and, after that, read more and more skeptical literature, however, still without publically talking about it. Only later, already teaching at the university, he let skeptical and parapsychology-critical topics become part of his teaching routine and began to do research in that field himself, which brought him nationwide recognition through a number of television appearances. As in the case of Hayley Stevens, his view on paranormal beliefs has become more tolerant over time. He now stresses that not all psychics are frauds, but some are simply victims of self-deception, and that not all belief systems that are almost certainly wrong have to be harmful, for example if people find solace in the belief in life after death. Also, he appreciates that, while the phenomena looked for by parapsychology very probably don't exist, the majority of the people doing research there does good scientific work, from which one can learn much about the psychology of beliefs and perceptions, but also about methods and mistakes in other fields of the social sciences [8]. Chris French's process of changing his mind was quick and basically complete after reading just one book, but he now puts it into the perspective of a personal development that has lasted for decades and still continues today. In the decisive step, personal discussions didn't play a role, but the systematic presentation of skeptical arguments in the form of a book did. Probably the special situation plays a role that for him the relevant information and arguments before that book and before the internet, simply weren't accessible without lengthy, targeted research. In addition, for the young Chris French, his belief in the paranormal was much less a part of his identity than it was for other people we have interviewed.

Breakdown and a New Sense of Happiness

Probably the most prominent British psychologist who has turned away from the belief in the paranormal is Susan Blackmore who is otherwise most known for her work on the theory of memes (ideas that reproduce and evolve like genes). During her college years, she had an intensive out-of-body experience, the perception of leaving her body and seeing it from outside. Today she explains that experience with sleep deprivation and drug use, but at the time she saw it as proof of a soul existing independent of the body and for the existence of a whole spectrum of paranormal phenomena. *"And at the age of 19, I had this wonderful idea that I would prove to the world and to all the narrow-minded scientists that were teaching me at Oxford that there were other worlds that they ignore."* As there was no funding available for such a project, she had to pay for her own Ph.D. research. While the general sentiment in her subject at the time was purely behavior-oriented and against her topic and her assumptions, Susan Blackmore only recalls one person she had controversial discussions with: A tutor at the university, whom she had told about the fresh impression of her out-of-body experience, simply recommended she should stay away from drugs. Later, the same tutor would also try to convince her of a more conventional doctoral topic. That tutor was not successful, as Susan Blackmore not only fought her way through her thesis in parapsychology, but also until today is a fervent supporter of the use of cannabis. Her doubts about parapsychology finally came from the results of her own work: The more soundly she set up and evaluated her experiments about telepathy, clairvoyance and other suspected phenomena, the more the initially encouraging results dissolved into thin air. At the same time, she found that other parapsychologists had more rigorous theories than she had - but also had no sound experimental evidence to show. *"I remember the moment when I thought: What if none of it works? I remember it so clearly. And then it all came crashing down."* That that moment only came after 5 years of mostly single-handed work doesn't irritate her one bit: "Oh, that was really fast. I definitely wouldn't have wanted it any faster. It took time, and it took that emotional involvement, and it took a lot of thinking and hard work." When she had almost given up the hope of finding actual supernatural phenomena, she got the opportunity of cooperating with a much more experienced experimenter, who had spectacular positive results to show. Her mixture of admiration and doubt turned to shock when she found that he probably manipulated his results himself, but at least was highly negligent in preventing manipulation [9]. Today she sees herself as belonging to the skeptic movement and has written books about how out-of-body experiences can be created in the brain.

> I want to share that joy I find in scientific understanding with people who so far don't want an explanation because they think they have to be mysterious and believe in souls and spirits to adequately honor their experiences.

In her long and challenging transformation process, discussions with the other side weren't important. Rather it was mostly driven by her own work, and finally by the betrayed trust in the work of some colleagues.

> **Food for Thought**
>
> When have you ever changed your mind an issue that was important to you? How much time did it take you? Can you name an experience or communication that was critical to that process? What was it about this experience that moved you? Was there anything someone could have said or done to make you more likely to take that step? How do you experience communication today with people who think the way you thought then?
>
> Please also feel free to share your experiences with us, as a personal message or as a comment on www.fakt-und-vorurteil.de.

3.5   A Sobering Interim Conclusion

So what can we learn from the biographies presented? The good news is certainly, first of all, that a change of mind is possible. It is rare, but it does happen again and again that people turn away from prejudices and turn to scientific facts, even if they have already made important decisions based on their belief and this belief is part of their self-image or even the source of their livelihood. It is striking, however, that all of the individuals considered here were still relatively young at the time of their transformation, in any case still in the first half of an average life span. The transformation processes were often painful, full of doubts and inner, sometimes also outer, conflicts, and they sometimes dragged on for years. In most cases, for very different reasons, a crack appeared in the system of faith, and it was in coming to terms with this initial doubt that the actual transformation took place.

What these biographies also show, however, is the limited role that discussions with representatives of scientific-skeptical thinking played in these transformation processes. All these people actually changed their minds themselves; as a rule, they were not persuaded by anyone or even taught better. In many cases, critical discussions did not even take place because there were no contact persons or discussions were unconsciously, and in some cases even actively, avoided. Relevant discussions also played a role at different stages of the transformation processes. In individual cases, as with the doctors Natalie Grams and Florian Albrecht and the Catholic skeptic, they played an important role in creating the first crack in the belief system that initiated the transformation. In the case of Britt Marie Hermes or Jessica Schab, discussions with skeptics only became conceivable late in this process and, above all, enabled them to arrive in a new social environment. The way in which these discussions proceeded also differed considerably: they ranged from understanding to informative to personally offensive and dealt partly with the content, but also partly with the conditions and consequences of faith. It is this aspect, namely the different ways in which such a discussion can be conducted, that we want to address in the following section.

Takeaway

Turning to scientific thinking coming from an irrational belief system is difficult. It requires self-conquest, the search for truth, and in most cases, a lot of time. Individual discussions and the rational arguments that are made can make small contributions at best. Ideally, they can nudge small cracks in the belief system, make the skeptical side look a little more competent, willing to talk, or friendly, or welcome someone already in the transformation process in what may initially be a frightening world of skeptical thinking.

The bad news is: the chances of making a difference worth mentioning in a single discussion are slim, and there is no magic formula. The good news is: Many types of communication can have a positive effect under certain circumstances. Sometimes it is the very polyphony of critics that leads to someone sowing that one seed of doubt that finally provides the decisive impetus.

References

1. Jeising T (2014) Irrtumslose Wissenschaft? Bibel Gemeinde 114(1):2
2. Warnke U (2011) Quantenphilosophie und Spiritualität. Scorpio, München
3. Hümmler HG (2019) Relativer Quantenquark, 2. Aufl. Springer, Heidelberg
4. Schmied B, Betsch C (2019) Effective strategies for rebutting science denialism in public discussions. Nat Hum Behav 3:931–939
5. Webster R, Marshall G (2019) The #TalkingClimate handbook. How to have conversations about climate change in your daily life. Climate Outreach, Oxford
6. Hermes BM (2019) Justice prevails! Cancer quack Colleen Huber loses her defamation suit against me. https://www.naturopathicdiaries.com/justice-prevails-cancer-quack-colleen-huber-loses-her-defamation-suit-against-me/. Accessed on: 4. März 2020
7. Haberlandt S (2017) Ex-Verschwörungstheoretikerin: Was hier passiert, ist Gehirnwäsche. https://noizz.de/politik/eine-aussteigerin-aus-der-verschworungs-szene-im-interview/7x50l23. Accessed on: 12. März 2020
8. French C (2018) Reflections on pseudoscience and parapsychology: from here to there and (slightly) back again. In Kaufman AB, Kaufman JC (Hrsg) the conspiracy against science. MIT Press, Cambridge, S 375–391
9. Blackmore S (1987) A report of a visit to Carl Sargent's laboratory. J Soc Psyc Res 54:186–198

4

Basic Strategies

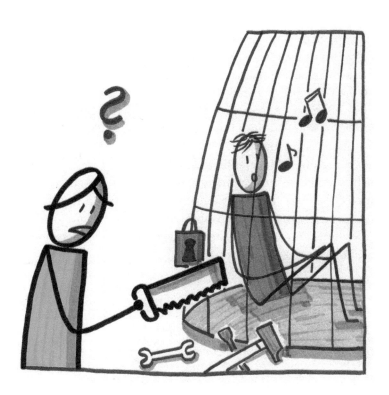

H. G. Hümmler, U. Schiesser, *Fact and Prejudice*,
https://doi.org/10.1007/978-3-662-66032-4_4

If a sufficiently large number of scientifically skeptically thinking people discuss with each other, then it is usually only a matter of time until the conversation turns to the perceived fact that "the other side" simply communicates better. One should not rely on the persuasive power of factual arguments, it is then often said, because one is not dealing with a knowledge deficit among the believers. Instead, one should argue more emotionally and, for example, focus on the touching individual fates of patients in alternative medicine. Similarly, the demand is repeatedly made that skeptics should deal with the other side in a more appreciative and understanding manner and take their concerns seriously.

If one imagines the actual implementation in practice, it is not difficult to see that these goals are at least partially in conflict with each other. For example, it is problematic to focus on individual failures of alternative medicine if, at the same time, it has to be made clear that individual cases do not allow any conclusions to be drawn about the benefits that can realistically be expected from a therapy. It is generally a problem to convey scientific findings in an emotional way if one wants to show that it is precisely the goal of the scientific method to avoid emotional distortions when gaining knowledge. If one wants to follow the principle of taking the opposing side seriously, one must also restrain oneself from emotionalizing, and taking anti-Semitic or otherwise misanthropic positions seriously makes it difficult to meet their representatives in an appreciative manner.

Quite apart from the very different reports of our interviewees, it must therefore be stated that, from a purely logical point of view, there is no universally "correct" strategy for discussions with believers. So let us first look at different dimensions in which possible discussion strategies can vary. They sometimes sound similar and are not always completely independent of each other, but in any case they are clearly distinguishable.

4.1   Arguing Confrontationally or Sympathetically?

First of all, it may seem obvious that in a factual discussion it cannot be helpful to denigrate one's counterpart on a personal level. Getting personal can not only quickly end a discussion – but possible listeners or fellow readers will also recognize a so-called argumentum ad hominem[1] and hold it against the person making the argument.

---

[1] Argumentum ad hominem is the attempt to invalidate a statement by criticizing its author. On the one hand, this can be a logical fallacy, but on the other hand, it can also be a deliberate attempt at rhetorical manipulation.

In politics, it is usually considered an ideal to argue hard on the merits but fair on a personal level. Given the psychological effects described in Sect. 2.2 it can be extremely treacherous to follow this ideal in practice. The fact that one wants to distinguish between the factual level and the personal level, and possibly does so from a sober semantic point of view, does not mean that the addressee will understand it that way. If you want to refute a central conviction or even a set of beliefs of a person on a factual level, for example, you have to break through the person's confirmation tendency and trigger a cognitive dissonance, which in many cases will be perceived as an attack on the person. If one criticizes such a belief not from a substantive but from an ethical point of view, the danger that this will be understood as a (fundamental) criticism of the person is even considerably greater.

It is not without reason that training courses on appreciative or "non-violent" communication are very popular in many organizations. However, the principle usually taught in these courses, namely to formulate judgments only with explicit reference to one's own subjective feelings and needs, is difficult to transfer to discussions of the kind considered here. After all, the point is precisely that science is not or should not be subjective, and everyone can have their own values and opinions, but not their own facts.

Indeed, several of our interviewees report being impressed by the kindness and understanding shown to them by some skeptical interlocutors as part of their transformation process. These include, for example, former ghost hunter Hayley Stevens and former cancer healer Britt Hermes. Unsurprisingly, it is these skeptics who are shining examples for them, and Hayley Stevens today regularly engages in sometimes heated arguments with skeptics whose communication she perceives as pejorative toward believers. Because of this pejorative attitude, she often feels frustration about a skeptical environment with which she actually agrees in content.

> I do wonder if that's why I have more of a mixed following, people who believe in things that I openly criticize, because I don't attack them or their beliefs, I attack the ideas rather than them, and make more of a meta-point doing that.

From this she has also derived the basic strategy for her own educational work:

> I'm also more and more about a sympathetic demeanor: 'I'm not here to convince you, but let's take the scientific look for once, and you decide what you're going to do with it, but listen to it for once.' That's a good-guy strategy to get people to listen. If you're nice and friendly and engaging, people are more likely to listen.

Skeptics are often perceived as sharp and cynical and harsh. That's two fanatics fighting each other. One is a believer in science, the other in esotericism. We must not only be the ones with the better arguments, but also the nicer ones, the ones who are better listened to. It doesn't need every insult and joke from our side either.

Natalie Grams, a physician who used to practice homeopathy, recounts her first contacts with skeptics, singling out in particular Edzard Ernst, professor emeritus of complementary medicine at the University of Exeter (himself a believer in homeopathy in his younger years):

In the beginning, I did not dare to address scientists like Edzard Ernst. What surprised me most was how nice they were. How human, cordial. Edzard Ernst is a dear, kind-hearted person. Until then, I always thought scientists were ossified old farts in sterile laboratories. The fact that they were so nice and friendly and eager to teach me something helped me lose my shyness. I thought, "Hey, you can totally talk to them, they're just normal people, they're not evil at all, they're not paid and biased."

Such an understanding approach is not always easy, however, when, for example, children are harmed by beliefs in quackery or the Holocaust is justified by conspiracy myths. Nor is it necessarily the only path that can lead to success. Both the skeptic with the religious belief in miracles and the physician Florian Albrecht, for example, report that their transformation processes began with being challenged aggressively and sometimes very personally in online discussions. In their case, it was apparently their efforts to defend themselves against such harsh criticism that led them to look into the topic more intensively and also to inform themselves more. As a believer in conspiracy, Stephanie Wittschier was not amenable to her family's attempts at understanding conversation. Today, she advocates drawing a very clear line against conspiracy thinking and runs a Facebook page which takes on the conspiracy scene not only with information, but very often also with ridicule. Psychologist Sebastian Bartoschek has taken to intentionally insulting people, at least online, if they already start the discussion with personal attacks against him – prepared to end the conversation at that point. *"Then some of them get to the point where they realize, okay, maybe that was too much, maybe what I did there was just crap."* That can sometimes be a new entry point into a meaningful dialogue, he says.

With regard to the severity of the confrontation, even people who have already been on the other side prefer very different strategies depending on the case, although friendly, appreciative communication is likely to be preferred by the majority.

4.2   Actively Present Your Own Arguments or Reactively Refute Those of the Other Side?

Closely related to the question of how confrontational one enters a discussion is whether one argues more actively or more reactively. Hayley Stevens cites an online discussion with a skeptical participant on a portal about ghost sightings as an important contribution to her transformation process. Her counterpart did not attempt to provide evidence that ghosts do not exist or even to convince her that the ghost image she presented as evidence showed something entirely harmless. Instead, accompanied by a brief explanation, he proposed the pareidolia described in Sect. 2.2 as a conceivable alternative explanation. The careful argumentation allowed her not to feel attacked by the critical interjection, and at the same time, it aroused her curiosity. As a result, she began to recognize more and more supposed ghost photos as pareidolia.

In the debate about clearly harmful forms of alternative medicine, such as the toxic chlorine bleach ingested or used as enema under the name MMS, it is not very effective to refute only the claims about the alleged benefits of the remedies. Instead, one cannot avoid at least pointing out their dangerousness, which is otherwise usually concealed or downplayed.

Based on the philosophy of science, skeptics in discussions about paranormal phenomena could basically retreat to a purely reactive argumentation. After all, a proof for the non-existence of such phenomena cannot be provided in principle – for example, try to prove once that the earth has never been visited by extraterrestrials! Rather, the one who claims such paranormal phenomena, from ghosts to an effect of homeopathic high potencies, is under the obligation to present evidence for his claim. Simply pointing out this burden of proof, however, is itself again part of an active argument.

4.3   Clarify the Facts or Evaluate Morally?

From a purely scientific perspective, it seems obvious that a discussion should be conducted on the factual level, separate from moral judgments. In practice, of course, such a value-neutral stance is not always easy when, for example, one finds that parents make their children victims of medical charlatanry or when pseudoscience is combined with racism.

Some of our interview partners also found their way out of anti-scientific belief systems precisely by morally confronting their own actions. Jessica

Schab, for example, did not question her role as an Internet guru until she became aware of her responsibility for the mental health of her followers. Among her former followers, she notes that rational approaches are partly rejected on principle: *"Feeling is more important, the right method. Thinking is seen as the wrong method. Thinking has an unpleasant association, as if you offend them when you confront them."*

For Britt Hermes, it was the conceivable punishability of her alternative cancer treatments that led her to the first critical research. At the same time, she emphasizes how relieved she was that the first skeptics she then contacted did not reproach her.

Here we see the fundamental problem with moral considerations in such discussions: It can be very helpful for people stuck in unscientific belief systems to think about the ethical consequences of that belief – but it is usually unhelpful to be reminded of them by others. Thomas F., a pediatrician who used to believe in homeopathy, reports from his current work about a completely failed communication with vaccine-critical parents: *"That was certainly my problem, that it went wrong because I was annoyed. I then said, 'That's totally selfish what you're doing.' The mother just cried, and the father might have been open in principle – but not after that."*

4.4   Discussing on the Factual or on a Meta Level?

Moral evaluation is not the only way to leave the purely substantive level in a discussion. In principle, that's what the aforementioned online discussion partner of ghost hunter Hayley Stevens did when he talked in general terms about the phenomenon of pareidolia, rather than engaging in a discussion of what might be discernible in a specific image. Educating about perceptions and self-deceptions gives a sincere believer the opportunity to question his or her own positions, which bypasses much internal resistance.

In the case of conspiracy believers, one could instead address why we all have a tendency to believe in unprovable conspiracies: they follow the principle of grasping our environment in patterns, replacing coincidence and uncertainty behind spectacular events with correspondingly spectacular explanations, attributing abstract threats (for example, from a virus) to concrete culprits – and they are also usually just good, exciting stories.

An interesting topic can also be what function a particular belief fulfills for someone. Criminal psychologist Lydia Benecke refers to a discussion she had with a right-wing populist who had made hate comments about her on Facebook for what he thought was justifying criminals. *"Looking at his profile, I noticed that he was mourning his childhood and had a totally unsuccessful current life."* When she approached him about it, she was initially met with astonishment, *"But the funny thing is that he then went into it and said, 'Yeah, I'm unhappy and talking about how shit all the refugees are right now because I'm not doing well,' and got to the point of saying, 'Maybe I should go to therapy and think about myself again.'"*

If it is not possible to credibly distinguish these fundamental considerations from the individual question, however, there is also a danger that the counterpart will not feel that his or her argument and, if applicable, his or her concern are being taken seriously. In the worst case, this discussion strategy can also come across as lecturing and condescending.

4.5 Presenting Arguments as Statements or Asking Questions?

A relatively common recommendation for discussions with believers is to ask critical questions rather than formulate factual arguments oneself. Among other things, this is supposed to help avoid the implicit personal attack through a substantive contradiction or to give the counterpart the opportunity to recognize the shortcomings of his argumentation himself.

The extreme form of this approach might be the discussion technique of *Street Epistemology*, which was developed by the American philosophy professor Peter Boghossian specifically for the purpose of converting people to atheism [1]. A substantive argumentation is completely avoided and the believer is instead repeatedly asked which method he used to reach his conviction and why he considers this method suitable. The answers are summarized by the questioner and used as a basis to ask for the next justification. Critics of the method complain that it challenges the rhetorical ability to clearly formulate and justify one's own position rather than the belief's content that should actually be criticized [2]. Especially in the case of a clear intellectual gap, there is also the danger that the believer feels rhetorically outsmarted and even less taken seriously.

The psychologist Sebastian Bartoschek did his doctorate on conspiracy thinking and has had positive experiences with asking questions to conspiracy believers in order to break through entrenched patterns of discussion. He reports on a discussion with a denier of the legitimacy of the German government whose demands unmasked themselves after a few queries: *"Chancellor Merkel must go? Who then is to become chancellor? Oh, the German Reich continues to exist. And who then is the rightful emperor? A Staufer, like in the middle ages? That's for the people to decide? In what form of government?"*

Since questions, if they are not merely rhetorical in nature, evoke less emotional rejection than direct contradiction, it is quite conceivable that such an approach can reach people and make them think who would not be at all amenable to normal argumentation. On the other hand, there is the danger that listeners or fellow readers who follow such a conversation may perceive the way the conversation is conducted as manipulative or even get the impression that you are only asking questions because you have no arguments yourself.

4.6   Arguing Soberly or Emotionally?

Giovanni Trapattoni was not a fan favorite after FC Bayern Munich hired him as coach for the second time in just a few years. The club's supporters were less than enthusiastic about the reserved, aristocratic-looking Italian, who usually spoke publicly through interpreters. That changed on March 10, 1998, with a single press conference after an embarrassing defeat against FC Schalke 04. Trapattoni's angry speech in clumsy German made him arguably the most popular soccer coach in Germany; his phrases "weak as bottle empty" and "I have done!" found their way into popular culture as idioms. What outstanding successes as coach of several clubs had failed to achieve, a moment of honest emotion did.

Conspiracy believers would never be swayed by facts because it felt better to remain among like-minded people and consider themselves superior, argues Mikhail Lemeshko, a physics professor from Vienna who is highly committed to didactics. The positive emotion outweighs all facts [3].

The journalist Sebastian Herrmann advises in his book "Starrköpfe überzeugen" (Convincing stubborn people) to tell good stories with simple contexts, to connect one's message with positive feelings and to rely on the "emotional force of the individual case" and avoid statistics [4]. This is problematic for the representation of scientific points of view, because in order to avoid subjective biases in science, it is precisely solid statistics that are decisive. On the other hand, only existential statements ("There is one …") and no generalizations ("For all … applies …") can be derived scientifically from individual cases. Thus, science can at best illustrate its results with emotional individual cases, but not substantiate them.

Emotions only work in a discussion if the addressees can empathize with them. Trapattoni's outburst of rage about his supposedly lazy big earning pros hit, possibly completely unplanned, exactly the nerve of many fans. Five years later, national coach Rudi Völler, who was actually much more popular in Germany due to his successes as a player, railed against critical sports journalists in a similar tone after the national team's 0–0 draw against Iceland, and this was predominantly perceived as primitive and embarrassing.

Representatives of scientific viewpoints are also often accorded less emotion in public than other participants in the discussion. In 2007, the science journalist Joachim Bublath found himself in the talk show "Menschen bei Maischberger" as the only voice of reason between the UFO-believing punk holdover Nina Hagen, parapsychologist Walter von Lucadou, esoteric author Johannes von Buttlar and angel therapist Sabrina Fox. When Bublath left the live broadcast prematurely after bizarre insults by Nina Hagen ("alien creature"), he met with applause and understanding in skeptic circles, but was also seen by others as a spoilsport or sore loser. The newspaper *Süddeutsche Zeitung* described Bublath's departure as "delicate in effect": *"Bublath appeared more confident when he simply smiled away Nina Hagen's alien hypotheses."* [5].

Food for Thought

Briefly visualize the last situations in which you had to discuss with believers from a scientific perspective. How do you classify your strategy pursued there in the dimensions mentioned here? What would your argumentation have looked like if you had chosen the other variant in each of the dimensions? How might the discussion have gone?

At the next opportunity, observe the strategies of the disputants in discussions on the basis of these dimensions. Who seems to you to be successful with which strategy? How do you experience the effect on yourself as a viewer/co-reader?

In sum, then, there is no really clear preference for a particular discussion strategy in any of the dimensions considered. So how you discuss with people who reject scientific findings depends on the situation, and before we pick out specific situations as examples in Part II, we will take a brief look at the systematic nature of such situations.

Takeaway

There are no fundamentally right and hardly any fundamentally wrong conversation strategies. A conversation strategy must fit the situation – but it must also fit you; otherwise it is not authentic. Sometimes the best strategy may even be to end the conversation.

It is therefore all the more important to clarify for yourself which strategy you are actually following and what alternatives there are. One can be more or less confrontational, more proactive or more reactive; one can discuss factually or morally, on the substantive level or on the meta-level, make statements or ask questions, and proceed soberly or emotionally. If so far you have not reached the other person at all, you should perhaps simply approach the conversation differently.

References

1. Boghossian P (2013) A manual for creating atheists. Pitchstone, Durham
2. Eponym (2019) Against street epistemology. https://www.lesswrong.com/posts/tb3mti2Y5znK5vs4L/against-street-epistemology. Accessed on: 1. Juli 2020
3. Lemeshko M (2020) Warum wir Verschwörungstheoretiker NIE umstimmen werden. Was machen wir falsch? https://www.youtube.com/watch?v=oNV_QR-Iej8. Accessed on: 13. Juli 2020
4. Herrmann S (2013) Starrköpfe überzeugen. Rowohlt, Hamburg
5. Kortmann C (2010) Ausweitung der Fluchtzone. https://www.sueddeutsche.de/kultur/tv-eklat-bublath-und-hagen-bei-maischberger-ausweitung-der-fluchtzone-1.327851. Accessed on: 15. Juli 2020

5

With Whom Do You Discuss and for What Purpose?

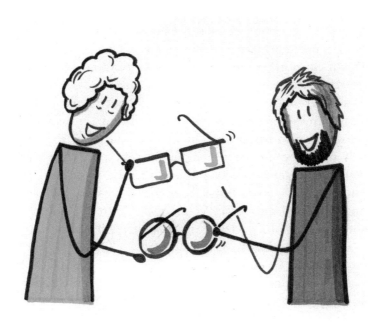

Which strategy is most likely to achieve something in a discussion with believers – and what is realistically achievable – depends on a variety of factors. These certainly include one's own knowledge and the purely objective provability of one's own position. However, the fact that this is not necessarily decisive in many cases has already been shown in the previous chapters. So let

H. G. Hümmler, U. Schiesser, *Fact and Prejudice*, https://doi.org/10.1007/978-3-662-66032-4_5

us first look at some quite different factors which characterize such a discussion situation and which can be decisive for its course:

- **The emotional relationship:** To a person who is close to us, with whom we have a basis of trust and an emotional bond, we have a completely different approach than to strangers on the Internet. Avoiding emotional conflicts by simply ignoring factual arguments is more difficult when they are made by a person who is emotionally close. Ignoring this close person ultimately also triggers a conflict. This effect works both ways, of course: To even contradict the deep convictions of a cherished or even beloved person is challenging and can become a serious burden for the relationship – however untenable these convictions may be from a scientific point of view. At the same time, the emotional closeness in the discussion also limits the means: Ending a dispute that has drifted into the pointless by referring to Tommy Krappweis' song titled "Entdumm dich!" (Unstupid Yourself!) is less likely to be an option vis-à-vis one's own parents or spouse than vis-à-vis a faceless pseudonym on the Internet.

- **Agreement on other issues:** There is some tendency for someone who recognizably believes in some unscientific concepts to be more inclined to believe in other unscientific concepts as well. For example, there are strong statistical correlations between beliefs in different conspiracy myths [1]. Psychologically, this is explained by more fundamental attitudes that are relatively stable over time, for example, the concept of transliminality [2]. This is the willingness to equate things that are consciously perceptible with things that are not. Ultimately, however, there are different facets in every person – and thus always commonalities. In 2020, Ronald Engert, the editor-in-chief of the Hare Krishna-affiliated magazine Tattva Viveka publicly distanced himself very clearly from COVID trivialization and conspiracy beliefs [3]. Around the same time, author Holm Gero Hümmler received encouragement in response to a critical blog article about a popular anti-vaccination activist from an alternative medicine practitioner who treats "traumas in mother karma" with meditation on ancestresses. And even while Theresa Stange strongly opposed vaccinations as a young mother, she would never have taken homeopathic globules. "*I think there's more that people have in common, people who believe in the paranormal and people who don't believe in the paranormal,*" former ghost hunter Hayley Stevens also explains. "*People who believe in the paranormal hate fraudulent psychics just as much as people who don't believe in the paranormal, and people who believe in lake monsters hate people who hoax monster photos just as much as skeptics do.*"

- **Power imbalance and responsibility:** Since a discussion takes place between human beings, it is practically never exclusively about the matter at hand, but always also about being right, and often about very specific decisions with which individual interests are connected. These interests can also simply include the affirmation of one's own autonomy, up to and including the "right to be unreasonable." The coach and theologian Peter Modler shows in his book "Mit Ignoranten sprechen" (Talking with igno- ramuses) how many discussions, especially in the professional environ- ment, tend to have the character of power games rather than the character of a meaningful weighing of arguments. Particularly when discussions revolve not only around abstract content, but also around concrete deci- sions, one must always keep in mind who can ultimately make these deci- sions. However, being able to make a decision also entails responsibility. This can become particularly apparent if the other party is a minor himself or if one of the parties bears responsibility for (possibly even joint) chil- dren. A very similar situation, and thus a very similar responsibility, arises when a party to the discussion, even without being able to decide anything directly, is in a role model position – for example, as a prominent artist or athlete. On the one hand, this responsibility is an all the more important reason to consistently look for secure information, such as scientific find- ings – but at the same time, it is more likely to lead to inhibitions among many people to pursue an overly confrontational discussion strategy.

  A special form of responsibility is felt by people who have set an example in their faith. *"As a spiritual leader, you're not allowed to change,"* former guru-YouTuber Jessica Schab recalls of her transformation process. *"They were very mad at me, my followers. They said I was a traitor and evil and brainwashed, I'm a part of the Illuminati. I constantly get letters from people who have just discovered my old videos."*

- **Personal relevance of the topic:** Practically everyone who represents scien- tific positions in social networks has had experiences with trolls who, for the sheer pleasure of provocation, make unsubstantiated claims, present quotes from supposed authorities taken out of context, and argue against straw men.[1] The most nerve-wracking thing about such contemporaries, however, is that they are usually quite indifferent to the actual subject of discussion, as long as they get the last word. As someone who cares about a topic, you then discuss it with someone who follows the pure pleasure of

---

[1] A straw man argument is a bogus argument where you impute an easily attackable statement to the other person that they did not even make. Thus one foists the assertion on homoeopathy critics that a homoeo- pathic treatment is ineffective, if they actually only point out that the globules administered thereby are placebos.

provocation. But one should not forget that one has a rather similar effect in the opposite direction if one discusses with a purely intellectual interest in a topic (because one knows, for example, that the claimed effect of "quantum healing" is physical nonsense) with someone for whom exactly this topic is a purpose in life (because he or she is convinced to have cured a large number of sick people for years with exactly this method). In the family, for example, it can also be extremely important for someone to want the best for the health of their children, even if, objectively speaking, they achieve exactly the opposite by wanting to "protect" them from the supposed dangers of vaccination. What for one person is a matter of science, truth, or simply pointed intellectual argument may well be a central aspect of self-image or economic livelihood for someone else.

It gets downright problematic, if, as psychology professor Chris French points out, one criticizes from a scientific, skeptical perspective, ideas that give someone stability in life: "Such situations are difficult for skeptics, because often, we attack some cherished belief, a belief that gives someone great solace. Sure, one can say, one should learn to cherish the beauty and greatness of scientific understanding – but not everybody can do that." Therefore, he held back his comments when the son of a university employee wanted to undergo mistletoe therapy as the last hope in uncurable cancer.

- **The chance to retreat:** Quite soberly, one has to state already at this point that in very many conversations of the kind under consideration, there is not the slightest prospect from the outset that one of the participants will convince the other. Theoretically, in such cases, one should spare oneself the whole discussion and simply let the other side believe. However, it may be that, as in the example of Sophie's mother in Chap. 1, one has to at least try to prevent someone from harming oneself. In such circumstances, one's retreat is blocked by one's responsibility for somebody else. Likewise, it happens – at grandma's coffee table or on the Internet – that you have a discussion forced upon you that you cannot escape without losing face. This can also apply to both sides: Who doesn't feel like having a discussion, won't always get a realistic chance of avoiding it.

- **Listeners and fellow readers:** When one thinks about the loss of face in the event of a refusal to discuss, one usually thinks less about the spurned discussion partner than about third parties listening or reading along. This is not only about one's own reputation, but also about the matter itself: If a confidently presented assertion remains unchallenged, it strengthens its credibility – even with listeners who would usually be more inclined to reject it. Under certain circumstances, you are no longer arguing for your counterpart, but actually only for the listeners or fellow readers. This is particularly important if you are not just any discussion participant, but are possibly perceived by others as a role model. However, it can also be important for less exposed fellow readers to show face and civil courage by taking a stand, for example in the case of inhumane statements.

- **Other social aspects:** Other people do not only have an influence on the course of a discussion if they are directly listening or reading along. The social environment has a great influence on belief systems and on the ability to let them go. If, as in the case of the former cancer healer Britt Hermes, practically the entire social environment consists of believers, then people discuss far more than scientific facts. The social context thus also has an effect on the personal significance of the topic.

This brings us to the next point: How promising different discussion strategies can be depends not only on the situation, but also on what one would actually consider success. The answer to what one aims for in a discussion with believers is less obvious than one might think at first glance:

- **Convincing the other side:** In her interview with us, the former conspiracy believer Stephanie Wittschier calls every discussion a "total waste of time" in which she does not succeed in getting a conspiracy believer out of the scene. In her position, with her high time commitment, her experience and her direct personal access to the scene, such radical expectations for her own success are quite understandable. For someone who is drawn into such a discussion rather unprepared and who has no personal connection to the counterpart, such expectations are very likely to end in frustration. But you don't necessarily have to set the bar that high.
- **Creating a crack in the system of thought:** The worlds of ideas with which one has to deal as a campaigner for scientific thinking are often closed systems of thought designed to exclude contradictory arguments. Only the believer himself or herself can break free from such a system of thought – but this presupposes a first crack, the recognition of a first contradiction or a first resistance to the values within this system of thought. "*The problem is, you have to get a crack in this bubble so that fresh air can get in there,*" pediatrician Thomas F. describes his first steps away from the homeopathic belief of his student days. As in his case or in the case of parapsychologist Susan Blackmore, this first doubt can arise from one's own failures, or it can be triggered by the behavior of other believers, as it happened to Theresa Stange, the vaccine-critical mother, or to conspiracy believer Stephanie Wittschier. But it can also be stimulated by thought-

provoking impulses, as in the case of ghost hunter Hayley Stevens, or provoked by contradiction, as we saw with alternative medicine believers Natalie Grams and Florian Albrecht. But such an outcome can hardly be foreseen or even planned. The seeds of doubt that can be sown are more likely to consist of many individual grains, where one never knows whether perhaps one of them will thrive.

- **Encourage an ongoing transformation process:** In the case of Natalie Grams and of former cancer healer Britt Hermes, but also in the case of psychologist Sebastian Bartoschek, who was originally a believer in conspiracy, it becomes clear how vital support is once a transformation process has begun. "*Can I think of who I am without my beliefs? This is hard for a lot of people who are believers. Because they are so sure they and their beliefs are the same thing, but they're not,*" Jessica Schab explains. "*It's just not like crafting a new identity – it's just shedding the layers.*" Those who radically turn around have a lot of questions, need a lot of information they've never sought before – but most importantly, they need confirmation that there is a life and a social environment outside the bubble of believers. However, it is not necessarily always obvious that someone is already in such a transformation process: Theresa Stange explains, for example, that it was precisely her growing insecurity about the anti-vaccination scene that led her to want to appear all the more convinced and self-confident to the outside world, and that she initially sought confirmation above all else.

- **Setting an example for listeners or fellow readers:** Listeners and fellow readers have already been mentioned, and even if a discussion seems completely pointless with regard to the other side, it can be an important goal to state one's arguments or simply a general objection for these seemingly uninvolved parties. This may even be necessary if the assertions made seem harmless at first glance. "*When does come to irrational beliefs, or even prejudiced beliefs, nobody just believes only in ghosts or just believes in psychics or just believes that they have to save the white race,*" explains former ghost hunter Hayley Stevens. "*Many British ghost hunting teams have Facebook pages where they post about their ghost hunts, but also, they'll post a lot of nationalist stuff on there.*"

- **Saving face:** If you have to worry about not being able to withdraw from an obviously pointless discussion without losing face, your only goal may well be to make a semi-dignified exit so you can then use your time more productively.

- **Achieve acceptable behavior:** If someone refuses to follow elementary hygiene rules in contact with others during an epidemic because that person is convinced the disease is faked by a conspiracy, then it may be neither possible nor necessary to convince them. At least in the short term, it may well be a sensible goal merely to change this person's behavior – if only because otherwise there is a threat of a fine. This is especially true when discussing with minors or when the goal is to protect children.

Food for Thought

Return to the situations you thought of at the end of Chap. 4. How would you characterize these situations in terms of the dimensions mentioned at the beginning of this section? Which of the stated goals did you pursue? Could others have been relevant?

Despite all the focus on one or more of these goals, one thing should not be lost sight of: In the end, it should not be about achieving one's goal at any cost and only through the better rhetoric rather than the better arguments. If you only "win" a discussion by presenting the stronger emotionalization, the more dramatic anecdotes, and the more entertaining story, you run the risk of ending up becoming what you actually want to fight.

Takeaway

When choosing a meaningful discussion strategy, it helps to be clear about who you're actually talking to and what you're trying to accomplish. Depending on the common ground you have with the other person, the situation you find yourself in, and the importance you attach to each topic, very different goals can be realistic. It does not always have to be about convincing the other person: Sometimes it is much more important to first set an example for third parties or simply to achieve that someone abides by rules, if necessary even without being enthusiastic about them.

References

1. Bartoschek S (2017) Bekanntheit von und Zustimmung zu Verschwörungstheorien – eine empirische Grundlagenarbeit, 3. Aufl. JMB, Hannover
2. Hell W (2010) Von Schafen und Ziegen. Skeptiker 2:56–61
3. Engert R (2020) Revolution, Diktatur und Verschwörung – die spirituelle Szene auf politischen (Ab-)Wegen. https://ronaldengert.com/2020/08/01/revolution-diktatur-und-verschworung-die-spirituelle-szene-auf-politischen-ab-wegen/. Accessed on: 20. Sept. 2020

Part II

Typical Discussion Situations

In this part of the book we finally come to the concrete recommendations on how to communicate with people who adhere to irrational belief systems. Since the conditions for such conversations can vary widely, as we saw in Part I, we consider different situations in each section. We encounter irrational beliefs particularly often in online communication, especially in social networks. This is simply because we encounter a particularly large number of people there and they talk about topics that they would only talk about with a select group of people in real life. However, very special conditions apply in online communication, and very special problems arise. While it is possible to simply break off many discussions online, this is hardly realistic in the family and among close friends. Here, conflicts are always particularly about the relationship between the people and about dealing with each other with understanding, reflecting on one's own role and keeping in mind that there is more at stake than just being right. At the same time, this tolerance definitely reaches its limits when the well-being of children is at risk. On the one hand, children can become the target group for irrational belief systems, but they can also be affected by the beliefs of their parents or others in their immediate environment. Conflicts between fact and prejudice, however, also occur in professional environments, for example in the workplace, and here both in dealings among colleagues and in relationships with superiors. Such discussions are no less problematic in medical or other therapeutic contexts – and here both the person offering and the person receiving therapy may have irrational ideas.

6

Many Things Are Different on the Internet

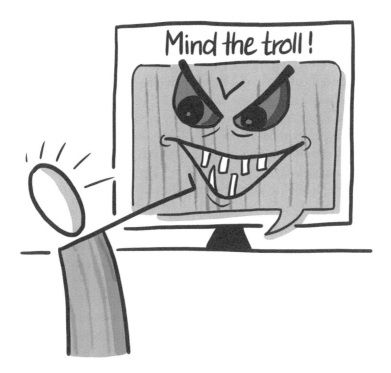

H. G. Hümmler, U. Schiesser, *Fact and Prejudice*,
https://doi.org/10.1007/978-3-662-66032-4_6

In the late 1990s, I (Holm Gero Hümmler) had my first experience with online discussions as part of an international particle physics experiment. My working group was based in Munich; the experiment itself and a large part of the scientists involved in setting it up were in New York and the rest of the researchers were spread halfway around the world. Video conferencing was still out of the question, international phone calls were still considered expensive, and the budget for air travel was limited – so communication was almost exclusively via e-mail, which most people had no experience with in their private lives. The developer of the database in which the many terabytes of measured data from the experiment were to be stored – and almost the only person who could answer technical questions about it – was Pavel, a Russian-born employee at the experiment in New York. For our team, which had experience, if any, only with the significantly different database structure of experiments at CERN in Geneva, Pavel's terse answers to our questions, in sometimes somewhat bumpy English, were a constant annoyance. My often impatient inquiries, usually copied to my Munich colleagues, were met with testy replies. Pavel became the bogeyman of my entire work group, without any of us ever having met him. Even a crisis discussion on the phone initiated by an experienced colleague did little to change this. A year and a half later, during an extended stay in New York, I once again had a problem with the database. I asked an American colleague for advice, and his first reaction, to my horror, was: "*Let's go see Pavel.*" So a few minutes later, somewhat unwillingly, I found myself standing in front of Pavel, whose office there was only one flight of stairs away from mine. In a huge cloud of cigarette smoke, I found a short, somewhat rotund man with a distinctive voice and a broad, friendly grin. After 10 minutes, Pavel had not only answered all my questions, but had also given me a set of useful tips on how to use the database – as well as a good dose of his irony-laden Russian humor. Later, back in Munich, my colleagues must have wondered why I suddenly got along so well with Pavel.

This very subjective story from the early days of Internet communication reveals some typical effects that still cause problems today, even in discussions with believers. Online discussions force the entire communication into a written form, whose immutability and quotability make it impossible to overlook irritating content, as one might do quite automatically in a direct conversation. In this written form, the entire framing of statements by nonverbal communication, which otherwise accompanies our personal statements, is also missing. Likewise, we lose non-verbal (and possibly also verbal) reactions of the recipient, which otherwise could help to recognize and eliminate misunderstandings or unexpected conflicts at an early stage. The practical reason that writing simply costs time may also lead to a more concise presentation in which one's own motivation is presented in less detail than in a personal conversation. Depending on the culture, an expected introductory small talk is sometimes also significantly more difficult.

These more difficult conditions make it much harder to really get to know someone as a person with whom you are only communicating online, which also makes it problematic to build up at least a basic mutual trust. For the chances of success of an online discussion, therefore, the question of whether you are having it with someone you have known before or with someone who is a complete stranger is quite crucial.

To make matters worse, there are forms of online communication that take the complications already arising with email to the extreme. Twitter, in particular, forces an even greater abbreviation of statements than already occurs through the written form. "*The bottom line is that no meaningful discussion can take place there; it's an exchange of individual sentences, an exchange of phrases, more of a self-promotion platform than a discourse platform,*" comments Austrian online journalist Sophie Niedenzu. Where longer texts would in principle be possible, it is often the use by mobile devices with their unwieldy text input function, especially with messaging services such as WhatsApp or Telegram, that leads to shortened statements. In the case of platforms such as Instagram or TikTok, which are strongly geared toward disseminating images or films, the user interfaces in some cases push the texts into the background to such an extent in comparison to the media that this alone makes it difficult to engage in a meaningful exchange of ideas. "*The statements are getting shorter, are less reasoned and are reduced to buzzwords,*" says Sophie Niedenzu. In networks without the obligation to use one's real name, but even more so in image boards and comment columns where input is possible without a fixed registration, the feeling of anonymity can lead to disinhibition, making discussions even more difficult. Finally, in the case of the majority of these platforms, it should be noted that the operators profit from the most intensive use possible with rapid interaction, because many page views increase advertising revenues. So every user is at the same time a part of the product for other users. To this end, portals such as Facebook or YouTube create an environment that encourages strong emotionalization, so that objectivity is particularly difficult to maintain there. The different, and in many cases more problematic, culture of discussion in these media is often accompanied by a culture of outrage going overboard. As a result, tolerating criticism or dissenting opinions tends to become the exception. In some cases, even small deviations from norms, even norms that were completely unknown to the offending person, lead to shitstorms, massive accumulations of negative comments and letters, which subsequently easily become insulting or threatening. In the case of shitstorms against companies or politicians, it is often difficult to tell whether they are a spontaneous wave of protest or an orchestrated campaign.

Food for Thought

Can you remember the situation in which you first became aware that completely different communication problems can occur on the Net than in normal life?

So, to account for these factors, you have to differentiate between certain types of situations also in online discussions.

6.1   Discussions with Strangers in Social Media or Comment Columns

Discussing in a social media portal or in the comment column of an online medium with a person you otherwise don't know at all pretty much brings together all the aforementioned obstacles to meaningful communication in one situation. The situation is not much easier with Facebook "friends" whom one knows only online and possibly only under a pseudonym. Here, we first consider the situation where the other person has made their position public either as their own post or as a comment on a third party's post. One is not necessarily addressed as a person and has the possibility to stay away from the discussion without exposing oneself. The situation where one's own statement on a blog or in a social network is attacked by someone else is then dealt with in Sect. 6.2.

In addition to the restrictions already mentioned for online discussions, in this case there are also the problems that there is no emotional relationship with the other person to build on, and that the situational factors listed in Chap. 5 are partly unknown. These include, for example, the personal significance of the topic for the counterpart, social aspects or his perceived chance to withdraw, i.e. whether he subjectively sees the option of avoiding the discussion. When someone spreads a conspiracy myth on Facebook, it is often not discernible whether there is a current insecurity behind it, a long-held belief system or pure pleasure in provocation. It is also not clear whether this person is supported in this belief, criticized or even ostracized because of this belief by those around him in his real life. Thus, it is often difficult to assess whether this person will drop out of the discussion when faced with criticism, show willingness to reflect or develop missionary zeal.

The first question in this situation is whether it is worth getting involved in a discussion at all, which of course depends on the prospects of success on the one hand and the possible damage to be prevented on the other. In the case of the prospects of success, there is also the question of what could be considered a success. The chance of actually convincing someone is even more slim without a personal connection than it already is in other cases. Saving one's own face is also ruled out as a necessity to participate if one is not directly addressed. It is also unlikely that someone who is already in the midst of a transformation process and is seriously interested in information will broadcast this uncertainty to the world on social networks or in public online comments. As far as the counterpart himself is concerned, the best that remains is the small hope of creating a crack in his belief system, which in the long term may create doubts and perhaps enable him at some point to break away from his previous ways of thinking.

Probably the most important reason for not ignoring unscientific or anti-scientific statements in social networks or online comments and for sometimes entering into a discussion after all is referred to in psychology as the illusion of truth effect: If you repeat various statements to subjects different numbers of times, they will tend to find the statements they have heard most often more credible than others [1]. This effect is independent of the age of the subjects [2] as well as of intelligence and thought styles [3]. If scientifically untenable statements are regularly left uncontradicted, there is a danger that uninvolved readers will increasingly believe them to be true.

Even those who disseminate such content themselves will, under certain circumstances, interpret the absence of contradiction as tacit approval. Even supporters of extreme outsider claims, such as the QAnon myth with its savior figure Donald Trump, like to see themselves as representatives of a "silent majority" [4]. This also explains that after two demonstrations against the Corona measures 2020 in Berlin, conspiracy believers spoke of more than one million participants, although calculations on the basis of aerial photographs came in each case to between 20,000 and 40,000 participants, depending on which rallies happening on the side were counted in.

Particularly when a belief system has a high potential for causing harm, there are therefore good reasons why such statements should be contradicted. This can be assumed, for example, if someone writes about the intention to take dangerous quack remedies such as the chlorine bleach MMS or to discontinue vital medicines such as insulin. Under no circumstances should one remain silent if children or other vulnerable persons are affected by such dangerous alternative healing methods. It is probably less dangerous if someone comments on zodiac signs for entertainment, associates their yoga classes with exaggerated health expectations, or takes Bach flower rescue remedy for their own peace of mind. Conspiracy myths, on the other hand, may not seem dangerous to the individual, but they are always a threat to democracy: the expectation that one cannot participate in shaping a society because it is controlled by sinister forces leads, at the very least, to a failure to make meaningful criticism and improvements. But often it also leads to political extremism – and in the worst case to hatred and violence.

In such cases, it is therefore important to make it clear that there is dissent and that this dissent is not an unsubstantiated expression of opinion by an individual. However, as the examples of the former ghost hunter Hayley Stevens and the physician Florian Albrecht, who has been cured of alternative medicine beliefs, show, it is still difficult to foresee in this situation which discussion strategy is helpful – after all, it is not even really clear what a realistic aim can be. Apart from the fact that getting too personal could get in the way of a later dialog, you can't do too much wrong at this stage. At the same time, the probability is relatively high that you will not achieve any discernible effect at all with such a comment. It is therefore generally not worthwhile to spend a lot of time making unsolicited detailed comments. A good approach is, for example, to cite fact checks or other critical articles as recommended reading without positioning oneself too clearly on them. In some contexts, uncommented linked articles are considered impolite and sometimes even deleted by moderators. In these cases, it usually helps to just briefly present the content and relevance of the source. Under certain circumstances, however, it is sufficient to start with a clear disapproval, without already building up your own argumentation, for example in the form: "*This is a conspiracy myth.*" Specifically for the case of hate speech in social media, the initiative "I am here" offers training on how to respond respectfully but clearly to such statements and also arrange to do so with like-minded people.

If you have decided to react to a statement that someone has made online and neither the person addressed nor like-minded people respond to it, then it is usually pointless to start a digital one-way communication with the person. The impression that you are harassing someone will not win you sympathy either from the person themselves or from fellow readers. If other discussion participants on your own side react, then it certainly makes sense to also answer their questions or clarify misunderstandings. However, there is little point in getting involved several times in an onslaught of comments from one's own side. On the contrary: if, for example, someone receives several hundred negative comments in response to an outrageous statement, then it is more likely to diminish the impression they make if it quickly becomes apparent that the same commentators appear in them again and again.

If, however, one receives responses to one's own comment from the person addressed or from their peers, then the perspective changes, and one is challenged to react to that. This brings us to the topic of the following section.

Food for Thought

Be honest: When did you last have the feeling that you absolutely had to convince someone who had spread false claims on the Internet?

6.2   Public Comments on Your Own Posts

If you've written posts on the web yourself that are commented on, or if you're directly approached about your own comments, you no longer have the option of simply staying out of the whole situation. Even if you do not comment, you must expect that this silence will also be interpreted as a comment. Before we turn to online discussions with known persons in Sect. 6.3, however, we will continue to assume that the person challenging us in this way is someone unknown.

Thus, the situational factors addressed in the previous section remain unknown, although the statement that challenges us to respond may already allow us to draw some basic conclusions about the situation and intentions of the other person. In order to be able to arrive at a meaningful strategy, it is advisable to strive for a preliminary classification of the counterpart into one of five categories on the basis of this statement, possibly existing background knowledge, the reactions of third parties and, if necessary, the early continuation of the conversation.

The Curious Person

In the case of the curious person, the unscientific position he or she holds has not yet become an element of a closed world view. It could be, for example, someone who saw a dubious report about a conspiracy myth on late night TV yesterday and is still under the fresh impression of the arguments put forward there. It can also be someone who has had a positive experience with an alternative medical treatment for the first time.

Curious persons do not necessarily identify themselves as such, but may well make provocative statements. However, they often react in a less missionary or aggressive manner to queries or contradiction than true believers who see their worldview questioned. Curious people also often have less factual knowledge about a topic than others who have been building their worldview on it for years. They are therefore more amenable to fact-based arguments, especially since they are basically still in the process of testing relatively newly absorbed information for its reliability. They may even react, perhaps only secretly, with relief to a well-founded debunking to the ideas they have just adopted, which may still be a little scary to them themselves. At the same time, they are often not yet familiar with the controversies that arise with the topic. Aggressive or emotional contradiction can therefore more easily upset or anger them and lead to a non-scientific position being perceived, if not as factually well supported, then as more likeable.

A good first approach in dealing with potential curious people is therefore to provide factual information on a generally understandable level, which can also be presented with some restraint, for example as a reading recommendation. Since even those interested in conspiracy myths generally do not yet reject all "mainstream media," articles from major newspapers or news magazines as well as contributions from reputable television formats are suitable, especially fact checks directed at a broad audience, such as, in German, on tagesschau.de.

If you're ready for a little more personal involvement, you can also try unexpectedly direct approaches to get around the problems of online communication described at the beginning. Florian Aigner, who docs science communication for the Vienna University of Technology, reports on Twitter [5]:

> Just got vehemently attacked online. Googled the gentleman, found a cell phone number and called. Quickly agreed, now we are friends. The Internet makes us all worse people than we otherwise actually are. Let's talk to each other!

If, in the course of the discussion, you find that you are not dealing with someone curious after all, you can always switch to another strategy.

The Believer

Believers do not believe *that* a certain facts are true – rather they believe *in* these facts. In this regard, the sentence of countless Sunday sermons applies to true believers even outside the church: "*Faith is more than knowledge*," as also stated in the Bible's Letter to the Hebrews, unconditionally "*not doubting what is not seen*". This, of course, is in blatant contradiction to the principles of scientific thought, which include that one can only arrive at better knowledge by being willing, at least in principle, to cast doubt on all knowledge. Accordingly, true believers in a discussion are often not concerned with the exchange of facts and opinions, but above all with proselytizing for their faith.

So in discussions with true believers, all the psychological factors that were shown in Chap. 1 work against you. By criticizing beliefs, one almost inevitably attacks the person of the believer, plus, in many cases, large parts of his social environment. If, in addition, this person is unknown, then, according to everything we have seen so far, it is very likely that one has no chance of convincing him. Thus, the only realistic goal with regard to this person is to possibly create a small crack in their belief system, which could possibly be at the very beginning of a longer transformation process. In this case, one will probably never know about a positive result sometime in the future. So there is something to be said for not wasting time on such a discussion. In this case, however, we are dealing with another conceivable target group, namely the people reading along.

Of course, there may also be believers among those readers, as well as people who are curious or who have started to doubt, and who can possibly be reached at least to some extent with good arguments. Above all, however, there may be people among them who have not yet formed a final opinion. Many of them may also have a scientific point of view, but are uncertain or looking for arguments. Especially for these people it would be particularly problematic if the wrong statement would stand uncontested. Then the already mentioned illusory truth effect, according to which even wrong statements are believed, if only one repeats them often enough, could unfold its full effect. However, one does not have to deliver scientific elaborations with data and references for the fellow readers nor to get involved in a detailed discussion with the believer: Basically uninvolved people often do not even invest the time to follow such argumentations. What they will – and should – remember is simply the fact that there has been a reasoned or even just a general objection. In addition to a general statement, it may be worthwhile to give a brief explanation of why one will not participate further in a continuing discussion. This should also largely avoid a loss of face to the outside world.

The Troll

Unlike a true believer, a troll is not primarily interested in proselytizing, but rather in having the last word. He does not discuss for something, but against someone and likes to use provocative or destructive lines of argumentation. A troll can be a believer at the same time, in the sense that he is actually convinced of the contents he represents – however, this is by no means necessary, and the difference is often only noticeable when one encounters the same person in discussions again and again, and he takes possibly contradictory positions. In any case, the motivation is not proselytizing for a belief, but the pleasure in provocation.

The main person responsible for the skeptical GWUP blog, journalist Bernd Harder, reports comments on a blog article recommending a podcast about nuclear energy. One commenter accused the blog of, "*once again advertising atom power.*" The commenter had obviously not been interested in the recommended podcast at all – otherwise he would have noticed that, despite the relatively neutral announcement, it was critical of nuclear energy.

Contrary to what the name suggests, the provocation of trolls is by no means always clumsy, but can have the character of a sophisticated intellectual game. In any case, the main goal is to make the other person look bad. To this end, trolls like to use logically incorrect argumentation such as trick questions, black-and-white thinking, or appeals to seemingly unassailable authorities or to "nature." It is equally popular to make an assertion and demand that it be considered true until proven otherwise. A popular variant of this, especially in social networks, is the linking of YouTube videos, sometimes lasting several hours, to which a statement is then demanded, possibly with the announcement that the video contains new arguments that have never been heard before. If someone actually takes the trouble to watch the video and respond appropriately, then the troll can simply link the next video with a promise of even newer and more spectacular arguments. If you draw the troll's attention to the inadmissibility of his argumentation or explicitly refuse to respond to it, then you give him the opportunity to put himself in a victim role.

Obviously, it is futile to try to convince a troll. Even before the advent of social networks, when online discussions still took place primarily in forums and mailing lists, the phrase has therefore circulated: "*Don't feed the troll.*" Behind the recommendation not to feed trolls is the idea that responding to provocations of this kind only ever encourages new provocations. This is often the case regardless of whether the response is friendly, understanding, dismissive, or even aggressive: A troll will either continue to provoke or make accusations from the victim role. If, on the other hand, there is no reaction at all, a troll usually loses interest quickly.

However, the idea that trolls can simply be ignored is associated with several problems. For example, on public platforms with many readers, it cannot be assumed that all participants will actually comply. In addition, it is not necessarily possible to tell that a person is a troll before he or she enters the discussion, unless the person in question has already appeared in the same role on several occasions. Finally, similar to believers, there is the danger that a claim that is left unchallenged will be believed by fellow readers or will lead to damage to the image of the person being addressed.

If the troll comment refers to a post that you yourself have published, many online platforms offer you the option of deleting the comment and, if necessary, excluding the person from further interaction. If you delete the comment without effectively excluding the troll, however, there is a risk that he or she will protest against the deletion and thus make himself or herself out to be a victim. In addition, bystanders may notice the deletion, which can also create a bad impression. On the other hand, depending on the platform and the topic (from experience, most often on YouTube), it can happen that the level of discussion is so low and the density of trolls so high that it is sometimes better to prevent discussions from the outset and delete comments completely or not allow them in the first place.

It will therefore be necessary in many cases to explicitly declare a discussion with a troll to be over – at the risk of opening up a victim role for him again. If the person in question can be at least vaguely classified ideologically, you can try to take him or her to task for peace by referring to common values ("Don't we all want …"). Otherwise, the only thing that helps is a clear announcement.

The Bullshitter and the Tactical Liar

As we have already seen with the trolls, not everyone who spreads an unscientific claim is necessarily convinced of it himself. Under certain circumstances, such claims are also simply pretexts. This happens especially when scientific findings come into conflict with one's own values, ideologies or habits. Bullshitters and tactical liars differ from trolls primarily in that they are less concerned with provocation than with not being disturbed in their own convictions by troublesome facts.

For example, it may have been a pretext in many cases when long-time supporters of Donald Trump declared in January 2021, contrary to obvious facts, that the storming of the U.S. Capitol had been staged by left-wing activists. Nor will many a climate change denier really consider himself more competent than 99% of climatologists, but simply not want to change his behavior. The same applies to some self-proclaimed virologists in the course of the COVID-19 pandemic. Denying the dangers of the disease was simply the more socially accepted way of resisting potentially painful restrictions than demanding to ignore the health and lives of those at risk.

Perhaps it is no coincidence that many scientific works on such claims come from the country where Donald Trump would become president. Back in the 1980s, philosopher Harry Frankfurt coined the term *bullshit* for claims where the person making them doesn't care if they are true or false, as long as they are convincing enough [6]. Thus, the bullshitter does not even claim to have evidence for his allegations – verifiable facts are replaced by perceived truths. More recently, the concept of the *blue lie has come up*, which is based on the established English idea of the harmless white lie, which is beneficial to coexistence. A typical white lie would be, for example: "*Your boiled broccoli tasted very good, grandma.*" Blue lies also serve coexistence, but only within a group, while excluding and attacking other groups [7]. For example, the tale of leftist Capitol stormers was uncontroversial among many Trump supporters because it exonerated everyone from accusations of supporting an attempted coup and thus served group cohesion while attacking supposedly violent leftist anti-fascists.

However, distinguishing bullshit or a purposeful lie from a purposeful actual belief that is maintained, for example, because it reduces cognitive dissonance, is difficult. For people with whom one communicates only online and whom one may not even know personally, such a distinction will even be impossible in many cases. One must also be aware that a direct challenge in the form of. "*You don't believe that yourself!*" implies a massive personal attack.

What is important for online communication is above all that one will certainly not be able to convince someone who spreads claims that are very self-serving (or serving one's own group). This is ultimately true regardless of whether it is a self-serving belief, or *bullshit* or *blue lies*. The goal here must be above all to offer clarifying information for fellow readers. Pointing out the usefulness of the claims is a sharp rhetorical sword – but also a double-edged one.

The Transforming Person

People who are currently undergoing a transformation process like the ones our interviewees in Chap. 3 described are actually the most important contacts you can reach in discussions. They are looking for information – and often for a new environment that will accept them despite their new, more critical perspective. Accordingly, it would be particularly important for them to get help in accessing verified scientific facts on the one hand, and on the other hand to feel accepted and not rejected or laughed at because of their previous views.

At the same time, however, those in a transformation process will often be particularly reluctant to reveal themselves in a public discussion. There, they are not only exposed to attacks from formerly like-minded people who may regard doubters as apostates, but also have to fear ridicule from scientifically minded people. For example, former ghost hunter turned skeptic Hayley Stevens distanced herself from "the skeptic movement" again in 2020 because she experienced the demeanor of many skeptics toward believers as condescending and hostile [8]. For those willing to change their minds, the very expectation of ridicule can be extremely off-putting. Thus, former homeopathic physician Natalie Grams and former cancer healer Britt Hermes were downright stunned when the first skeptics they came into personal contact with after much hesitation turned out to be friendly, understanding, and helpful. It is therefore hardly surprising that Theresa Stange, as a vaccine-critical mother, took great pains for a long time to hide her uncertainty and to express herself as if she were a completely convinced anti-vaxxer.

Particularly in the often harsh tone on social networks, one cannot necessarily assume that people who are in the process of turning away from faith and toward knowledge will also identify themselves as such. They may well act as missionary believers or even as trolls in order to test the arguments, but also the personalities, on the previous "opposite side" and learn to assess them better. Yet, this is often difficult or even impossible to distinguish.

However, if you have clues that you are actually reading from someone who is in a transformation process or at least open to it, then you should offer this person as much helpful information and encouragement as you can. Dare to give the doubter the benefit of the doubt!

Food for Thought

The different types of discussion opponents are listed here for the case of online discussions, but of course you encounter them in real life as well. Try to find examples of the different types from conversations you remember well.

Let your examples sink in for a moment ... Honestly, how sure are you that you didn't make a mistake?

6.3   Discussion with Acquaintances on Social Media

If you are not talking to a stranger in such an online discussion, but to a person you have known for a long time, possibly in real life, then this person may of course also find himself in one of the five roles described. One should expect that the incentive for aggressive troll behavior would decrease among aquaintances, but the basic tendency to be right even on the most absurd topic is something that most people know even from their closest family and friends. Acting as a troll is not so much a personality trait as a social role one assumes in a particular context. However, it should be much easier to assess which of these roles a person should be assigned if that person is known.

At the same time, the option of not responding to an unscientific statement is significantly limited if this statement comes from a well-known, possibly even cherished person. If one is not addressed directly, ignoring can still be an option in principle. However, as soon as it is a matter of ideas that restrict freedom, socially exclude or even endanger health, one is more likely to feel the need to at least point out contradicting facts with acquaintances than with strangers. If, on the other hand, you are addressed directly by acquaintances in social networks, then ignoring or deleting the comment, as well as a brusque rejection, would in many cases be understood as an affront.

However, having a familiar person in front of the other screen in such a discussion also has advantages. For example, one's own arguments are less likely to be ignored or brushed aside by a known counterpart. The trust that we place in people we know in a positive sense is a connection and ensures that the counterpart will at least deal with the opposition in some form. But this, too, is a double-edged sword: The closer you are to someone, the more likely you are to regard objective criticism of a statement as an attack on your own person.

But there's another difference when communicating online with someone you already know, and it's almost always an advantage: It's much easier to move the discussion out of the public eye and onto a private communication channel. As a rule, that's what you should aim for, even if it's just the text messaging function of the same online portal. If the channel change succeeds, then we find ourselves in the situation that is already much more favorable for a productive exchange, which the following section deals with. If you have to assume that the public part of the discussion was followed by a large number of fellow readers, you should still let them know that the conversation is being continued in private (possibly also virtually) and has not been abruptly ended by one side.

If, on the other hand, the other person refuses to switch to a more private channel, or if he or she deliberately sought public discussion, even though we might have met in person in the near future, for example, then the question naturally arises as to why he or she attaches such importance to an audience. This could simply be trolling, but it could also be an attempt to keep the personal, non-public exchange free of controversial topics. Those who are unsure of their own position, which could be the case with curious or transitioning people in the system introduced above, may even feel safer in a public setting with many supposedly like-minded people.

Food for Thought

Think about people you regularly deal with both publicly on the Internet and in direct contact. How does their behavior differ in the different roles? Are they more professional, more distant, or more uninhibited online?

Do you know people who seem to embody completely different personalities in real life and on the Internet?

Psychologist Sebastian Bartoschek experiences this kind of divergence between online persona and real-life demeanor in himself when he encounters people who, up to that point, had experienced him primarily as a journalist and online commentator: "*People come to me and expect to meet an absolute asshole, and then realize at some point: He's not like that at all. No matter how I come across online – to myself, of course, I feel consistent.*" He attributes this primarily to his preference for sarcasm and irony, which are far more often misunderstood online than in direct exchanges.

6.4 Direct Online Communication with Acquaintances on Private Channels

If you communicate online with a person you already know and are on a channel without fellow readers, the conditions for meaningful communication are much more favorable than in the public sphere of a social network. Under these conditions, for example, many of the incentives that cause people to act as trolls in online discussions no longer apply. Of course, there may also be people in your circle of acquaintances who can't resist provoking out of sheer pleasure in provocation, even without an audience of any kind. However, these are rather rare, and in a personal context one usually knows this beforehand. In addition, in a dialogue one has the possibility to end the discussion or to demand a change of topic without creating a negative impression with third parties.

At the same time, it is easier for people who are just forming an opinion or are just beginning to break away from the belief construct to open up in a personal environment. Without fellow readers, the fear of showing weakness by expressing doubts about one's own position is reduced. Questions can play an important role in determining whether you are actually dealing with someone with an established belief system: On the one hand, you can relax the situation, avoid arguments, and learn more about the other person's actual beliefs by asking questions yourself. On the other hand, hidden doubts on the part of the counterpart are most likely to be expressed in questions. Those who really want to know something will sooner or later ask questions. Thus, in the case of Theresa Stange, a vaccine-critical mother, the first hints to her new partner that her convictions were not as solid as she wanted to show were the questions: *"If you had children, would you have them vaccinated? With all the recommended vaccinations? Why?"*

However, there remain the problems that always arise with online-only communication – and thus there are still enough triggers for misunderstandings. For example, even with people you know, it's usually harder to "read between the lines" in online communication because the entire nonverbal level is missing. The sheer time involved in writing, especially on the improvised keyboard of a smartphone, also encourages statements to become more concise, which makes it difficult to respond appropriately to more subtle statements or underlying emotional needs of the other person.

A good approach in such a situation can therefore be to shift the conversation to an even more personal level and pick up the phone, for example. If appropriate opportunities exist, it is also a good idea to postpone the topic to a later point in time over a beer – which is not necessarily to be taken literally.

As has been shown in the course of the COVID-19 pandemic, video calls and online conferences can also be a way to overcome the limitations of online communication to a large extent when face-to-face meetings are not realistic. Of course, even this is not a full substitute for a face-to-face encounter, but the ability to perceive facial expressions, gestures, and surroundings of the other person is once again a significant improvement over the telephone and can avoid many of the communication obstacles outlined here.

The more direct the contact and the more relaxed the situation, the sooner it will be possible to grasp what function a belief system has for the other person and to respond accordingly. Then it will also be possible to use many of the approaches among friends that we address in Chap. 7 for discussions within the family.

Food for Thought

Now think about people from your immediate personal environment with whom you regularly communicate via different channels (e.g., personal conversation, telephone, short message services, e-mail, letter …). For which content (e.g., emotional exchange, making appointments, humor …) do you prefer to use which channels with whom? Are there also people with whom you prefer to discuss very personal and emotional things at a distance?

What can you learn from this for discussions with believers?

6.5   Dealing with Hate and Threats

Anyone who regularly posts scientific content on the Internet and takes a stand on controversial topics such as esotericism or conspiracy myths will sooner or later become acquainted with hate messages. In their personal character and massively pejorative or aggressive nature, they are usually easy to distinguish from acceptable criticism of someone's behavior or from a dissenting opinion on the matter at hand, which should be tolerated in a sociopolitical discourse. Hate messages can occur both as public comments and as personal messages through private channels. Sometimes, even when they refer to content on the Net, they come in the classic form of mostly anonymous letters or phone calls. It also happens that attempts are made to denounce the hated target person to their employer or, especially in the case of the self-employed, to harm them through false online reviews. A creative, but no less unpleasant (and possibly even expensive due to fees) form of hate message, which author Holm Gero Hümmler recently had to experience, was regular transfers of penny amounts with spiteful subject lines to his account number obtained under pretext. If hate messages cannot be deleted simply by clicking the mouse, this can considerably increase the psychological stress to which one is exposed.

Hate messages in public channels are sometimes difficult to distinguish from troll comments – at least at first glance. However, the different intention becomes apparent after a reaction at the latest, because the authors of hate comments usually only try to act out their aggression and then end the contact relatively quickly – at least for the moment. In any case, they are not interested in an exchange of any kind, even if they repeatedly cover the same victim with hate messages. Trolls, on the other hand, try to engage the victim in a discussion precisely through their provocation, so that they can then continue to provoke steadily. A troll also responds to counter-arguments – but for no other purpose than to keep the victim in the discussion. He will therefore also make the introduction provocative rather than repulsive.

A subtly perfidious form of hate comment, which is, however, sometimes also used by trolls as an introduction, has the form: "*I have always admired you so far, but now I am deeply disappointed in you.*" Especially towards artists, the recommendation to rather concentrate on singing/acting/writing novels or similar in the future and to refrain from political or social comments often follows. If one has the opportunity to check this (for example, on fan pages in social networks), one usually finds no indication that the person in question has actually shown any interest in the supposedly so revered idol before. Obviously, the aim here is to trigger remorse about supposedly lost fans and to provoke a justification. In fact, however, such a justification is likely to be of little use – neither to a hater nor to a troll.

Various experience reports on how to deal with hate messages are circulating on the web, which are also often presented as recommendations, but in many cases are at least not applicable to everyone. The Austrian correspondent of the *Spiegel,* Hasnain Kazim, has written a book about how he responds to frequently racist or xenophobic hate messages in a pointed and humorous way [9]. Politicians such as Peter Tauber and Markus Söder have repeatedly resorted to reading out excerpts from hate mail in public. Martin Hoffmann, online journalist at the *Welt,* has researched and called authors of hate messages. Green Party politician Renate Künast even visited them at home in some cases. Both report that they have experienced mostly very meek people, some of whom have apologized. The time required for this is, of course, considerable. Whoever chooses this path must also reckon with the fact that, as has happened to Hoffmann in other cases, he will simply continue to be insulted on the phone [10]. Künast has also repeatedly been involved in legal disputes with insulters, for which many victims of hate will want to spend neither time nor nerves [11]. The strongly contradictory verdicts in Künast's lawsuits against several Facebook users, who had called her a "piece of shit," among other things, also show how great the courts' margin is when it comes to the criminal offense of insult [12].

Finally, it is important to realize that many recommendations for dealing with hate messages on the Internet, such as those found at the Amadeu Antonio Foundation, are directed at the moderators of portals and comment columns [13]. If they engage in a discussion with a writer of hate comments, they are still in a position of power to simply delete his comments and possibly even block him permanently. As a private person under attack, one has this possibility at most on one's own profile in social networks or in the comment section of self-operated websites. In addition, even freelance professional forum moderators should have at least some support from their employer in the event of legal disputes. You don't have that support as a private person either.

Therefore, there is nothing dishonorable about simply ignoring non-public hate messages. It might be possible to reach some of the writers and make them think with a surprising counter-action such as the house calls by Mrs. Künast, but the effort would be disproportionately high for most of those affected. One also owes no answer to the authors of insulting, racist, sexist or similar hate comments: by the way they formulate them, they themselves have decided that they do not want to engage in meaningful dialogue.

In situations that one can moderate oneself, such as one's own social media profile, one should also certainly consider simply deleting meaningless hate comments and, if possible, blocking the authors from further access. In many cases, the authors will not even notice this, because they often no longer visit a profile with statements that are unpleasant for them after venting their aggression. If the hate comments contain statements that can be answered fruitfully for fellow readers, then one can provide these answers – depending on one's own temperament also pointedly – and then hope that the original hate commentator will discredit himself for fellow readers through his own aggressiveness. However, this only works if you are in a position to delete at least further hate comments by other authors that may have been attracted.

On public pages that you cannot moderate yourself, it usually makes no sense for the person being attacked to argue alone against hate comments. In such a situation, you need help – ideally from the moderators of the page, otherwise from other users who show solidarity. As Sophie Niedenzu, for years a forum moderator at the major Austrian daily newspaper *Der Standard*, reports, in many large online forums, some with tens of thousands of comments, posts are primarily reviewed by semi-automated systems. Only comments that a self-learning algorithm recognizes as possibly containing aggressive wording, or links, are checked manually: "*No human can read all that*." This shows how important it can be to also stand by other users when they become victims of hate comments. Such support not only helps in the discussion: the site aktiv-gegen-digitale-gewalt.de also emphasizes the importance of emotional support and a sense of community when one has become the target of hate messages [14]. One way to get involved against hate speech on the net and to cooperate with others is offered, for example, by the initiative #IchBinHier (I am here). No-hate-speech.de is committed to combating specifically group-related hate speech and offers useful tips on how to deal with such public attacks.

Social networks offer the option of reporting content, including comments that are suspected of violating laws or terms and conditions, for review. For the event that violations have indeed occurred, a promise is made to remove such content. Content to be removed should also include (at least group-related) expressions of hate as well as threats. In the case of repeated or serious violations, creators can also be temporarily or permanently banned from the network. In practice, these mechanisms work to varying degrees, partly to do with the automated or outsourced processing of such complaints in low-wage countries, and partly to do with the sheer overwhelm of mass reporting of content that someone objects to solely on ideological or personal grounds. Facebook in particular is said to delete pictures of female breasts more reliably than depictions of violence or Nazi symbols [15]. Nevertheless, people should take the opportunity to consistently report public hate messages on these networks. This may not always lead to the immediate deletion of the content, but it does serve more than just the reassuring feeling of having done something: It can be assumed that users whose content is regularly reported by different people will be monitored more closely in the longer term and will eventually be blocked after all.

For criminally relevant forms of hate messages, e.g., defamation or incitement to hatred, there is of course also the possibility of a criminal complaint. Threats can also usually be reported to the police, although in Germany, the criminal offense of threat is only fulfilled if it refers to a specific, serious crime. This would be the case, for example, with a threat of rape. Less clear threats of the form "*We'll get you*," "*We know where your car is*," or. "*I know your employer*" therefore do not apply. However, they can and should also be reported to the police, because they can, for example, constitute a criminal insult, which is, however, only prosecuted at the request of the victim.

Women in particular are often the target of online threats of violence, which certainly has something to do with the fact that women are thought to be less capable of defending themselves, and also with the particular emotional impact of sexualized violence. The net activist Katharina Nocun and the psychologist Pia Lamberty report on a flood of rape threats after they critically examined conspiracy thinking in their (highly recommended) book *Fake Facts*. Criminal psychologist Lydia Benecke suffered a similar fate after giving an interview about the psyche of the perpetrator in a particularly brutal rape case. Various right-wing websites twisted her statements in the interview into false claims that she had justified the perpetrator and advised all women who are victims of rape to hold still. She responded resolutely to the subsequent rape and death threats against herself: "*Since I've blocked about 500 Nazis on Facebook since then, there's not much more coming.*"

Criminal charges can be filed at any police station. In Germany, an uncomplicated option, where a report should be routed relatively directly to appropriately trained officers, is offered by the online stations of many state police departments, as well as, for all German states, by the "respect!" reporting office of the Baden-Württemberg Democracy Center, which is also recommended by the Federal Criminal Police Office [16]. In the case of permanent persecution with hate messages, it may make sense to seek legal advice. Free counseling options as well as many references for further reading are available from the HateAid initiative at hateaid.org or for Austria from the counseling center Zara at zara.or.at.

Negative comments and insults unfortunately have a stronger effect on us than praise and applause. If among 30 feedbacks there are two negative ones, it is these that will stay in our minds the most and matter to us the most. Attacks always attract our attention more than support. Those who are frequently confronted with hate mail will acquire coping strategies over time, and a habituation effect will occur here as well. However, they do not leave us completely cold, and that is precisely the intended effect. The stress of aggressive name-calling, threats and devaluations of one's own person can also have a traumatic effect and should be handled with conscious counter-strategies.

Food for Thought

Think about situations in which you have experienced how other people have become the target of hate messages – people you know personally or complete strangers of whom you may not even have witnessed how they received these messages. How have you yourself reacted in the process? How would you have liked to react?

What experiences have you had with hate messages yourself?

Practical Tips for Dealing with Hate on the Internet:

- As soon as you take a position and express an opinion, there will be people who disagree with you. In a discussion culture that promotes extreme positions and ennobles outrage as the main instrument of debate, you will always have to reckon with aggressive confrontations as well. *"If you don't have enemies, you don't have character"* actor Paul Newman is reputed to have once said. *"If you want to be Everybody's Darling, you'll end up being Everybody's Idiot,"* as politician Franz Josef Strauß put it.

- Is there a point of criticism that is justified – even if it is made in an inappropriate form? To immunize oneself against any form of negative feedback would be to throw the baby out with the bathwater. Can I learn anything from the feedback? Did I express myself mistakably, did I make a mistake in terms of content, was my own tone acceptable?

- Don't give the person more attention than is appropriate. The triumph of hate commenters is in the emotional impact they make. It may help you to remember that it is often the impotent, frustrated outcry of someone who is not doing so well at the moment. You are just the wailing wall, the rock on which the wave breaks, and you don't have to react at all if you don't want to. Reinhard Mey puts it beautifully in his song "Mein Achtel Lorbeerblatt" about his critics: *"So I do what a tree would do if a pig scratched itself against it. And I consider what each has to say, and keep nice and quiet, and sit on my eighth of a bay leaf, and do what I want."*

- From the same song comes the line: *"And as long as I have a few friends left, my flag won't hang in the wind."* Who are the people whose feedback and backing are important to you, whose expert advice you value? Exchange ideas with these people when you are confronted with harsh criticism. Stay in contact and exchange opinions with other professionals when the attacks arise because of your professional activities.

- In psycho- and trauma therapy one often uses inner images to better process events, to activate resources and to better deal with fears. One of these images is the magic cloak. Imagine you go to a magic workshop and have a magic cloak sewn to protect you from attacks and a hostile environment. What color, what material, what cut do you choose? In your imagination, put the cloak on. How does it feel to wear it? What do you hear when you move? What does it smell like? Imagine what happens to attacks directed at you: Do they bounce off the coat, are they thrown back, is the energy of the attack absorbed? What effect does the coat have on the inside? Does it give you composure, courage, self-confidence? You could imagine, before you start reading comments or emails, to put on this coat. The more often you use this image, the more familiar it is to you, the better it can develop a protective function for you. You can also develop other images that help you build up a certain distance and protect yourself, for example, the image of a zoo: each comment corresponds to an animal that expresses itself in a friendly or hostile way, silently or loudly.

- Pay special attention to those people who support you, from whom you receive thanks and recognition. Respond to this feedback, but also reward the effort of those people who offer constructive criticism. Get emotional support from those around you when an attack, abuse, or threat hits you personally. Be comforted, but don't give the negative comments much more attention and consideration than the positive ones.
- Show support and solidarity when others are subjected to hate comments. Oppose hateful, denigrating statements, the building of enemy images and stereotypes, the slander of minorities, ethnicities, sexual orientations, religions or worldviews, toxic language altogether. Movements like "#IchBinHier" [17] want to promote digital civil courage.
- Don't be manipulated into responding in an aggressive, hurtful tone. If you do respond, it's better to do so in the way you would have liked. Shame your counterpart with explicit politeness.
- Even if you don't feel directly threatened, filing a complaint or reporting a hate poster can be useful to show people that they are crossing boundaries and that their action is unacceptable. By doing so, you also protect others and future victims.
- Is a direct threat being made? Do I expect the person to even take action? If a hate message is frightening, be sure to file a complaint – especially if messages are repeated and come from the same person. In all cases, document the messages, take screenshots, create a "toxic repository" email directory. Repeated messages can constitute "stalking"; documentation of the duration and extent of the messages is necessary for this.
- Also, give yourself time-outs, breaks, and safe spaces if you are subject to many attacks.
- If unsure, contact a counseling center sooner rather than later.
- The rise of conspiracy myths is contributing to the fact that journalists are increasingly seen as an enemy and are exposed to direct attacks in addition to increasing verbal violence. Be careful with personal information such as address, family background, etc. Unfortunately, measures such as blocking the disclosure of one's own address in the civil register and an editorial security concept make sense. Tips and addresses can be found, for example, in the "Guide for Journalists under Threat in Germany" [18].

Takeaway

On the Internet, communication is in many cases reduced to written messages, which are often also highly abbreviated. In addition, especially in social networks or online comments, there is extensive anonymity, which can have a particularly disinhibiting effect. Online communication therefore runs according to its own rules, and it has produced its own role models according to which people shape their behavior in the virtual world. In discussions with people known in person, it is often helpful to shift the communication to a more personal medium. Hate and threatening messages are a particularly problematic topic on the Internet. You might want to take a picture of the practical tips just listed for dealing with hate on the Internet and have them ready on your smartphone or computer for a critical moment.

References

1. Hasher L et al (1977) Frequency and the conference of referential validity. J Verbal Learn Verbal Behav 16:107–112
2. Fazio LK, Sherry CL (2020) The effect of repetition on truth judgments across development. Psychol Sci 31(9):1150–1160
3. De Keersmaecker J et al (2020) Investigating the robustness of the illusory truth effect across individual differences in cognitive ability, need for cognitive closure, and cognitive style. Personal Soc Psychol Bull 46(2):204–215
4. Müller M (2020) X22 Report vom 19.08.2020. http://qanon.at/2020/08/20/x22-report-vom-19-08-2020/. Accessed on: 16. Sept. 2020
5. Aigner F (2020) Bin gerade online heftig angegriffen worden. https://twitter.com/florianaigner/status/1305912388009549824. Accessed on: 16. Okt. 2020
6. Frankfurt HG (2005) On bullshit. Princeton University Press, Princeton
7. Smith JA (2017) Can the science of lying explain Trump's support? https://greatergood.berkeley.edu/article/item/can_the_science_of_lying_explain_trumps_support. Accessed on: 12. Jan. 2021
8. Stevens H (2020) Parting ways with the skeptic movement. https://hayleyisaghost.co.UK/parting-ways-skeptic-movement/. Accessed on: 16. Okt. 2020
9. Kazim H (2018) Post von Karlheinz: Wütende Mails von richtigen Deutschen – und was ich ihnen antworte. Penguin, München
10. Ufer G (2016) Meet your hater. https://www.deutschlandfunkkultur.de/umgang-mit-hass-kommentaren-meet-your-hater.2156.de.html?dram:article_id=372948
11. Evers A (2020) Hasskommentare: Künast gewinnt Prozess um falsches Zitat. https://www.e-recht24.de/news/strafrecht/12065-kuenast-hasskommentar.html. Accessed on: 26. Okt. 2020

12. Süddeutsche Zeitung (2020) Künast siegt vor Gericht in Hate-Speech-Verfahren. https://www.sueddeutsche.de/digital/renate-kuenast-beleidigung-facebook-kammergericht-1.4855652. Accessed on: 26. Okt. 2020

13. Baldauf J et al (2015) „Geh Sterben!" Umgang mit Hate Speech und Kommentaren im Internet. https://www.amadeu-antonio-stiftung.de/wp-content/uploads/2018/08/hatespeech-1.pdf. Accessed on: 26. Okt. 2020

14. Grieger K (2020) Was kann ich tun? https://www.aktiv-gegen-digitale-gewalt.de/de/hatespeech/was-kann-ich-tun-2017.html. Accessed on: 26. Okt. 2020

15. Bubeck S (2016) Facebook: Staatsanwaltschaft ermittelt gegen Mark Zuckerberg. https://www.giga.de/unternehmen/facebook/news/facebook-staatsanwaltschaft-ermittelt-gegen-mark-zuckerberg/. Accessed on: 26. Okt. 2020

16. Bundeskriminalamt (2020) Meldestelle für Hetze im Internet. https://www.bka.de/DE/KontaktAufnehmen/HinweisGeben/MeldestelleHetzeImInternet/meldestelle_node.html. Accessed on: 26. Okt. 2020

17. https://www.ichbinhier.eu. Accessed on: 16. Febr. 2021

18. Neue deutsche Medienmacher, No Hate Speech Movement. Broschüre: „Leitfaden für bedrohte Journalist: Innen in Deutschland. Zum Umgang mit Bedrohungslagen." https://www.neuemedienmacher.de/helpdesk/fileadmin/user_upload/20201209_NotfallKits_NHS.pdf, Broschüre „Wetterfest durch den Shit-Storm. Leitfaden für Medienschaffende zum Umgang mit Hass im Netz." https://www.neuemedienmacher.de/helpdesk/fileadmin/user_upload/Leitfaden_gegen_Hassrede_2019.pdf. Accessed on: 16. Febr. 2021

7

Discussions in the Family

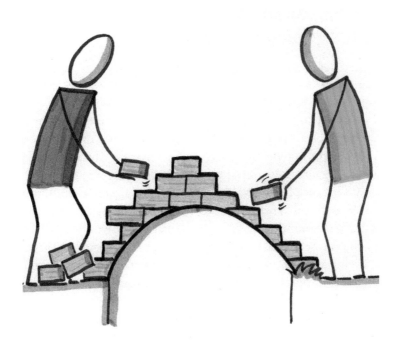

H. G. Hümmler, U. Schiesser, *Fact and Prejudice*,
https://doi.org/10.1007/978-3-662-66032-4_7

My mother has been diagnosed with breast cancer. She refuses to undergo the urgently advised surgery and chemotherapy. Instead, she wants to be treated in a dubious cancer clinic that works with questionable and unscientific methods. When I tell her my criticism, she starts to cry and accuses me of making it even harder for her and not supporting her. She says my doubt is like acid that hurts her aura and prevents healing.

***

My brother used the celebration of my 40th birthday to promote his dubious financial scheme to my friends. He has only recently become self-employed and is convinced that he will soon become rich with it. I think it's a pyramid scheme and don't want anyone else around me to get into it. When I warn people, my brother is pissed off and complains that I stab him in the back.

***

My new boyfriend grew up in a free church. His parents want me to come to services and expect me to be involved in church as well.

***

My ex-husband's new significant other claims to be a medium and to talk to spirits. Our children are 5 and 8 and were very impressed, but also a little scared by this. She told them that they are crystal children and all the things they have done in previous lives. I don't want my children to come into contact with this nonsense, but their father also seems to be getting more and more involved with esotericism.

Usually, we avoid contact with people who hold completely different positions than we do, be it in social values, politics, religion, questions of style or lifestyle. Our environment usually echoes our lifestyle. This is much harder to do in our family circle. In our circle of friends, we surround ourselves predominantly with people who hold similar positions to our own. In the family environment, political views, positions on religion and faith, and opinions on many topics are more broadly based. We can't easily avoid controversial discussions, but for better or worse are sometimes connected with people we wouldn't even exchange a word with on the street. And now we share vacations, holidays, important life events with the cousin who gives away cell phone stickers that are supposed to protect against dangerous mobile phone radiation; the sister-in-law who gives flaming speeches against vaccination at family gatherings and pulls out the appropriate globules for every illness; the great-grandmother who raves about her youth in the Nazi girl's organization and explains that Hitler had a good labor market policy and that the Holocaust never took place in this way; the parents who gleefully tell us that they want to invest money in a water treatment device that positively influences the vibrations of the water.

We are all familiar with debates and conflicts of different world views within the family circle. Family is exhausting, and that's a good thing! The culture of discussion has been declining overall in recent years; people are retreating more and more into ideological strongholds that are secured against any intrusion of foreign ideas. Black-and-white thinking and friend-foe images dominate the discourse. In the family, we cannot completely escape these conflicts. We have to listen to different points of view, formulate and argue our own. We have to tolerate other ways of thinking and living and find compromises together. We have to endure criticism of our cherished opinions and allow the seemingly self-evident to be questioned. Diversity is exhausting, but enriching.

7.1   Tips for the Conversation

It is necessary that you respect a person as a person, then you can talk to them. You can affirm and respect them as a fellow human beeing, that is the basis for a good conversation. (Krista Federspiel)

Key success factors that were repeatedly mentioned in our interviews are an appreciative approach and a good basis for conversation with the person you are trying to convince. Try to go into the conversation as a discoverer and researcher, not as a judge or teacher. If you only want to correct and instruct your relatives, you will appear as a fanatical zealot yourself. These conversations usually don't go far. Attacks on an important personal worldview are practically always seen as attacks on someone's person and trigger corresponding defensive reflexes. How often have you yourself changed your mind in the course of a discussion? We are not talking about trivial issues, but about important matters of faith, issues that affect your worldview, that are really important to you.

Food for Thought

Have you yourself once abandoned a fundamental political attitude, your religion, a socio-political conviction, your admiration for a role model, because of a good argument? If so, what convinced you?

What conversations can you recall that were important to your views? What in those debates influenced you?

What role did interpersonal relationships play?

We tend to follow people we value, who are role models for us, whose lives and attitudes impress us. *"We only learn from those we love,"* Johann Wolfgang von Goethe was already convinced of this. For conversations in our closest environment, this means that the relationship level is quite crucial if we want to reach a person. In families, which are in some ways involuntary communities, maintaining a good climate is especially important. We know that we're going to keep running into each other over the years. We have to have a certain amount of tolerance, even if our circle of friends doesn't usually demand it. When someone slips into anti-scientific or extremist ideologies, family can be a final corrective, an anchor, and a link to other worldviews that counteract the development of tunnel vision.

A key moment for me was a conversation with my sister. I asked her, "Does it actually bother you that I'm in Jehovah's Witnesses? Do you love me less because I'm a Witness?" And she answered, "No, I completely don't care. I will always love you, you will always be my little sister, and it doesn't matter what religion." That's when I realized that there is unconditional love. It wasn't like that with the Witnesses. With the Witnesses, my whole value was dependent on being in the community, on doing what they wanted me to do. That was an important realization. My sister and me did cool things together like shopping and going to a coffee shop, which you don't do in the Witnesses. I was able to talk to her about boys and learn about a different life. (Lisa L.)

Manipulating individuals and cult-like communities often try to isolate people from their environment as much as possible; contacts with friends are discontinued if they do not follow the new rules and views. In most cases, it is also recommended to break off contact with the family. Parents are denounced as the cause of all problems; contact with relatives is presented as harmful to personal development. Sometimes there is talk of "contamination" by negative energies that would emanate from relatives, especially when they speak out against involvement in the group. Friends who speak out critically are said to be avoided as "brakes" on one's own development. The more a person can be separated from his previous environment and integrated into a new community, the easier it is to control him, and the more the ideology solidifies.

If, however, there is a later withdrawal from this group, the family of origin is often a safety net, and sometimes it remains the only one of the social relationships that is not connected to the ideology. It can be a starting point for a reorientation, a bridgehead to free oneself from a repressive system.

My son told us parents that he had done a family constellation, and it had "come out" that we had never really loved him and were a harmful influence on him. He should free himself from us and therefore wants to break off all contact.

***

This psychic told my wife that she had been a priestess in a past life and I had been a crusader, and I had raped and killed her. She said that the two of us were karmically connected and would meet again in each life. My wife's task was to free herself from me. She should separate from me by all means. How can I defend myself against accusations that are not even from this life?

***

The preacher advised me to stay away from ungodly people. Satan would use them to cast doubt and lead me astray. Sin, he said, was contagious.

Create Good Conditions

Choose the place and time wisely: the more emotional a conversation, the more unpredictable. An outburst of emotion can help show the other person how you feel, how important or frightening a topic is to you, how great your concern. As a rule, however, such conversations are unproductive, can easily derail and have the opposite effect. The other person may be put on the defensive, statements are made in the heat of the moment that you later regret, and rifts are deepened. There is a danger that if you are highly agitated, you will not be able to listen at all and will resort only to primitive flight/fight responses.

It also makes little sense to assault your counterpart with fundamental questions about the relationship when he or she is on the run to work or has just come home tired. If three lively children are romping around you or the mystery novel is just getting exciting, the timing is also suboptimal.

Try to choose a good time and place to talk in advance. Where and when do the best conversations usually take place in your family? In the kitchen while cooking? While driving a car? When you're out for a walk? When you go out for a beer after a soccer match? Ask for a conversation and choose a good time and convenient place for it together. Conversations in pairs promote openness; more than two people can easily create the impression of a tribunal. However, a neutral third person can also be helpful in maintaining an appreciative, positive conversational atmosphere.

Cultivate a Culture of Discussion

We live in an age of outrage culture, and we are used to being outraged very quickly and radically rejecting everything that does not correspond to our own opinion. As a result, we then have no more room to differentiate between what does not correspond to our opinion and what is absolutely 100% dangerous and unacceptable. (Florian Aigner, science communicator)

Currently, sending links of internet sources often replaces the independent argumentation of a position. As many discourses have moved to online platforms, the logic and algorithms of the Internet are also changing the form of argument. Shortened attention spans lead to shortened positions. Emotion replaces arguments; thumbs go up or down. Attention is the currency of the information age, and extreme positions and polarization generate more attention. A common reaction to other opinions is indignation, anger and calls for boycotts. The position of Voltaire –. *"My lord, I do not share your opinion, but I would stake my life that you should be allowed to express it"* – has given way to a culture of outrage. Opposing positions are seen as an imposition, and moral superiority replaces debate.

In this book, we take the position that for satisfying conversations, your social skills are crucial, but the art of good debate also wants to be practiced.

The Information Duel

The following exercise is designed to help build communication skills and give both positions an opportunity to be heard in the same way.

Agree on rules beforehand:

- Make the topic more concrete: "global warming" or "corona" are too vague, and it is better to agree in advance on which aspect the arguments should revolve around. Perhaps formulate a question: what is the argument for/ against COVID vaccination? Can I get rich just by thinking/wishing in the right way?
- One person starts presenting the arguments. He/she is not interrupted and gets full attention. After fifteen minutes, the other person follows with his/ her own arguments.
- After the half hour, you go into free discussion.
- You can also put this on as a family show, hand out popcorn and have a group discussion or vote in the manner of a science slam.
- A very effective additional task can be to research the seriousness of your own sources and the quoted experts and present them to the audience before your own quarter hour. Each person chooses a maximum of three source materials (videos, books or websites) that he/she considers particularly relevant to his/her own point of view.

- Following the model of Anglo-Saxon debating clubs, it becomes particularly exciting when you have to switch roles and represent the other position.

If this format seems too involved, at least sit down together at the computer right away, instead of just sending links from videos and websites, and go through the material together. Check it with a timer so that each position gets the same amount of attention: for example, 10 min for the conspiracy theory video and then 10 min for the counter-post on Mimikama [1]. By limiting the time and dividing the attention fairly, it is easier for both sides to engage with each other's arguments. A lot of frustration in discussions arises from having the feeling that the other person is not listening at all.

7.2   Conversation Attitudes

Speaking in I-Messages

"I'm worried because …". You-messages are mostly experienced as an attack: *"You are not well informed," "You are making a mistake!"* Do not explain to your counterpart without being asked what he/she feels and why he/she acts the way he/she does: *"You let your guru talk you into everything because you don't want to make your own decisions and he is the good daddy to you that your own father never was!"* You may even be right with this statement, but the fine art is to say it in a way and at a time when your counterpart does not immediately feel attacked, basically deny everything and go into counterattack: *"You're just jealous and acting like a hobby psychologist, because now everything doesn't revolve around you!"* At this point, the conversation quickly escalates and veers to any couple or family conflicts that may already exist.

Better would be:

> My impression is that your guru is an important advisor for you. If you have felt well supported by him so far, it is also logical to seek advice from him for everyday problems, as some do from their own parents. I can imagine that it can be a relief to have someone you trust enough to leave some decisions entirely up to him. But your guru can be wrong, too. I don't trust him the way you do, and I worry that you rely on him too much and that his advice isn't always right.

A chain of reasoning of this form is also called a **Yes Set:** at least three statements that the other person can easily agree with or that express general facts are followed by the person's own concern. In this way, a positive connection and an automatic pattern of agreement are established suggestively. This sounds very manipulative, and it is. This method is used in sales, for example. But we can learn from it that it helps if a bridge is built first, before one's own arguments can have an effect.

Avoid Misunderstandings

Make sure that you have understood your counterpart. Summarize the arguments briefly. *"Did I understand you correctly: You are of the opinion … "*

You will be surprised how often misunderstandings happen in communication, how often you can only correctly reproduce a fraction of what was said. Our preconceived opinions and expectations serve as a filter that already takes effect in the physical reception of information. In short, we hear what we expect to hear.

> **Takeaway**
>
> Good arguments alone will not change anyone's mind who is getting emotional benefits from a worldview. As long as he/she gains security, support, and belonging from the belief, it will be maintained until there is a better substitute or a personal experience shakes the conviction. The influence of the environment often only has a long-term effect. It is important to stay in touch to prevent the relative from staying exclusively in an ideological echo chamber.

Understanding the Motives

It's not about knowledge, it's about feeling safe in a world that has become insanely complicated. (Martin Puntigam, Science Buster)

It is quite crucial to know the driving factors of your conversation partner. Not being dismissive is sometimes difficult; it helps to keep in mind what benefit an ideology has for the person. It helps to look at the roots of enthusiasm: What needs are being met? Ideologies are not free-floating constructs; they are based on needs, fears, desires, experiences. It can be a need for security, for belonging, for health, for meaning and purpose. If there has been a change in attitudes: What was important at that time in the person's life? Was there a turning point, a particular event that generated stress: a death, a separation, job loss, health or financial problems, a crisis of identity or meaning? If so, the person probably found satisfaction of needs, answers, and support in the new ideological home.

Based on the model of psychologist Hilarion Petzold [2], we can speak of five pillars on which our identity is based:

1. Body and health: self-image, sexuality, how comfortable I feel in my skin.
2. Social relationships: Family, friends, love relationships, colleagues, social network, society.
3. Work and performance: all activities, paid or unpaid
4. Material security: income, standard of living, perceived security.
5. Values and ideals: religious and political convictions, sense of meaning, art and culture.

Psychotherapist Sylvia Neuberger has used Petzold's model to develop a counseling tool for the field of cult counseling. She assigned the pillar "work" to the area of "material security" and instead dedicated a separate pillar to people's need for meaning in their actions, work and existence (Fig. 7.1).

For a stable personality it is favorable if all five pillars are well filled. A weaker pillar can also be balanced by the others; but if there are too many weak points in several areas of life, an imbalance arises, a deficiency that must be filled. This happens especially often in crisis situations, upheavals and new phases of life. Various groups and providers offer solutions for this. *"In this sense, the path into the so-called cult can be seen as an attempted solution to an existing problem."* [3] If these needs cannot be satisfied in any other way, an

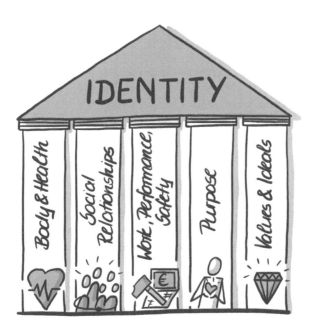

Fig. 7.1 The five pillars of identity according to the counseling model of Sylvia Neuberger

ideology is maintained with all its might, no matter how negative the consequences may be when viewed from the outside.

In counseling, with the person affected or, more often, with the relatives, they are asked to mark for each pillar on a scale of 1–10 how well (from the subjective point of view of the person affected) each need was met, immediately **before** the first contact with the problematic community. The next step is to assess the extent to which the membership in the group has filled these gaps: again, from the perspective of the affected person; the concerned environment probably assesses the benefit differently. To answer these questions, family members need to put themselves in the relative's shoes. This promotes understanding and ends the impasse of blame. When the motives for joining a so-called cult are clearer, the person's environment can also consider whether it can provide support in the underlying problem: What needs, worries, fears find an answer in the community, the guru, the ideology of their relative?

My partner is very afraid of getting multiple sclerosis like her mother.

***

My nephew is the only one in a family of academics who, after dropping out of his studies several times, has still not found a profession and lives on welfare and odd jobs. He is the problem child and black sheep of the family. Now he has discovered his vocation as a shaman and declares that a middle-class life would hinder him in his true task. Before, at family gatherings, everyone talked at him and gave him tips; now he wants to explain the world to us, lectures us and knows everything better.
***

My wife wants to give the children the very best childhood and spends hours surfing parenting forums to learn about vaccination. She is very concerned about doing more harm than good to the children by vaccinating them.

For better understanding and empathy, it is helpful to recognize in which area a belief is (seemingly) stabilizing. Perhaps this insight will also give you an idea or two where you yourself can help stabilize one of the pillars. With adults, of course, this is more difficult; you cannot solve life-tasks for another person. With adolescents, parents are very much co-responsible and also have more possibilities to influence. For example, they can be supportive if their child has little social involvement. They can support membership in clubs, sports clubs, positive circles of friends.

Sabine has recently been enthusiastically advertising in multi-level marketing for a company that offers natural cosmetics and nutritional supplements. The family is annoyed because sample packs are handed out at every meeting and they feel emotionally blackmailed into ordering the products. Sabine gets a surrogate family there, status, the hope of becoming rich, the belief that she is helping other people with the products, saving them, the feeling that she is doing good for herself and her body, and possibly even a surrogate religion. Why would she give that up? For what? And the more time, money and energy she has invested in it, the more unswervingly she tries to justify those costs *(sunk cost fallacy)*. No one likes to admit they were wrong. It triggers painful feelings of shame.

Don't focus too much on the content of an ideology in conversations, but pay attention to the motives: Why does someone believe something? What benefit is there in being a member of this group? What fears does the group address? What does it (seemingly) offer solutions for? What would the person have to do without if they left the group?

> *You can't let them dictate the topic of discussion. I don't talk to someone who is prejudiced against foreigners about foreigners. I talk to him about anything, but not about this. For example, someone grumbles about social parasites, "They do nothing and get everything, and I have to work." Now I can respond with statistics and say, look, this is what migrants pay in, and this is what they get out. It's also important to have those arguments present and to know that, but in conversation it's more important to have the ability to see what's behind those statements. The repressed desire to be lazy and taken care of. I respond, "When you say it like that, it occurs to me, I have a desire to be cared for like that too. How cool would that be, to not have to get up in the morning and to get everything served in bed." And you notice how the other person's eyes light up. Then we talk for an hour, not about social parasites, but about the difficulties in the achievement-oriented society, the elbow society, of dealing with such longings in a different way than suppressing and repressing them and then projecting them onto others. That's what I mean by the detour. There is no point in opposing on this other level.* (Andreas Peham, right-wing extremism expert)

Appreciation Through a Change of Perspective

How we evaluate behavior depends to a large extent on our frame of reference.

Even behavior that seems problematic to us can have a good intention behind it, and every characteristic contains positive as well as negative facets. In systemic therapy, this approach is called "reframing." We change the frame with which we look at a particular issue. This changes the meaning. The goal is to be able to look at a characteristic, a behavior from different perspectives and to perceive it in its diversity. Someone is fanatical? Then perhaps he is (at least in this area) also enthusiastic, passionate, consistent, persistent, tenacious, unbending, an idealist, true to his faith even against opposition. He is willing to swim against the tide, filled with the desire to create a better world.

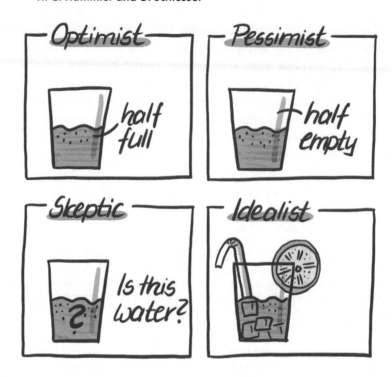

He stands up for certain people and causes, even if it means negative consequences for himself; he doesn't do things by halves.

Dare to change your perspective and try putting on benevolent glasses for once. This does not mean that you gloss over problematic ideologies. In most cases, we tend to choose the most negative interpretation anyway; positive reframing is much harder for us. Extremists and fanatics lack the will and ability to change perspectives and empathize sympathetically with others. It is easier to see oneself in the right and to reject the other person, the other position, on principle. Recognizing that the other person also has complex motives promotes dialogue.

My mother had no understanding for the fact that I dropped out of my studies and wanted to dedicate my whole life to my guru. I wanted to live a humble, deeply spiritual life, serving only other, socially disadvantaged people. We had a big fight about it, she criticized my guru, which I could not tolerate at all at that time. But she also said that she admired my social commitment, my courage to live my ideals so uncompromisingly and that she herself would also like to be so independent from the values and norms of our consumerist society. It was so important for me to feel understood by her here. The conversation was like a bridge between us. It helped me to turn to her again after I left the group.

This change of perspective enables us to find the "common ground", the things we still have in common. Where, despite our differences, are we similar in our views?

In the discussion with the uncle who suspects the conspiracies of the Freemasons everywhere, a unifying link can be that we both do not approve of secret collusion by the powerful and the rich for their benefit; that we both think that power needs control; that we both think democracy is very essential and want to protect it. What dangers threaten it and what protective measures we consider sensible may differ. But it is easier to accept different views when the basic values and concerns we have in common are identified.

> This makes it possible to label racism as such at the Christmas table with the family and to take a stand against it, but still try to move toward a common ground. How do you come up with that statement? For example, with right-wing narratives: We both think poverty sucks and think something should be done about it. (Fabian Reicher, Social Worker)

> ***

> You can have radically different opinions without questioning a person as a human being or your relationship to that person. (Florian Aigner, science communicator)
> ***

> Our neighbor has been going on and on about how he thinks "the foreigners" are social parasites. At first I put up with it, for the sake of good neighborliness, until it was enough for me: "I agree with you that a functioning social system is important and good. That must suck when you get a cancer diagnosis and can't afford the drugs. Imagine having to take on debt and think about whether it's going to pay off every time you go through treatment." He seemed surprised by this turn of events, and we were united in our horror at the idea. At his renewed reference to those he felt were abusing the system, I again agreed with him that people need to feel that equity prevails in the distribution of resources. Again, we agreed, and he shared with me how important the issue of justice is to him in general. In response to my objection that corporations that make a profit in Austria but pay no taxes burden the system to a much greater extent, he agreed with me, and we ended the conversation on a friendly note. After that, when he displayed prejudice on a topic, I would address him about not being fair in his judgment, then he would listen to me. We often disagreed, but with a little attention there was always a common denominator that allowed us to be reconciled in the end.

Humor

> What is your star sign? – I have resigned. (Evelyn Preis)

Humor is a strategy to cope with difficult situations. It relieves stress and is a positive resource. It can also serve as a test of fanaticism for communities and ideologies. Is it allowed to laugh about the content, the people at the top, the rituals and customs, or is it immediately considered an insult, sacrilege, disrespect? The ironic self-examination, the caricature and the joke create critical distance, put criticism in a nutshell and show us how small the distance is from the sublime to the ridiculous. *"Laughter takes the shiver out of the sacred,"* Hubert Schleichert formulates in his book "Wie man mit Fundamentalisten diskutiert, ohne den Verstand zu verlieren" (How to talk to fundamentalists without losing your mind) [4]:

> Ideologies of all kinds, especially religions, hate laughter because they know how dangerous it is. He who laughs at a thing is no longer afraid of it. [...] The fear of laughter is the fear of thinking.

If you are in a family, perhaps for years in dispute about an issue, the fronts are usually hardened, and a "tunnel vision" sets in that makes it difficult to move away from one's own position. Humor can ease tensions, lead to a different perspective and build bridges. It creates distance to the problem and can thus help to interrupt ingrained patterns of thinking and behavior [5]. Humor can help a skeptical-scientifically oriented person to endure irrationality, miracle addiction and esoteric excesses. Among like-minded people, laughing at the position of others unites them. In the exchange between different positions, however, you need tact and humorous talent to be able to use laughter as a bridge. A prerequisite is that you can also look at yourself and your own position from a distance with humor. Otherwise, you run the risk of coming across as cynical, insensitive or dismissive. Above all, avoid coming across as humiliating or shaming.

> Wit and humor will get you relatively far. You don't always have to crack the whip. Rather respond with humor and point out flaws in the line of reasoning. (Sophie Niedenzu, journalist)

> ***
>
> *The sarcasm, the exaggeration, the joke is of course something that also conveys an easier access to a topic. We know, of course, that when someone laughs, they are more accessible to information.* (Christian Lübbers, ENT physician)

Questions Instead of Preaching

> You have to be very careful not to get into that know-it-all role. In order for an argument to fit, I have to understand the life and way of thinking of my counter-

part, even if it is irrational. What makes this person tick? I have to hook into the worldview that people have, not start with mine. (Krista Federspiel, journalist)

Ask questions, and listen. Questions encourage your counterpart to look at their own attitudes. Changes in our attitudes happen only after changes in our views. An inner process must first be set in motion. Questions are more useful for this than sermons:

About the content and sources

- Where does this information come from?
- How trustworthy is this source? Why do you trust it?
- How likely is it that this information is true?
- Have you ever used a different source?
- What if you are wrong and it is not true?
- Who benefits from spreading this information?
- What would have to happen to make you change your mind? How would I have to convince you? What arguments and evidence would you accept?

About personal experience

- Have you ever had this happen to you?
- How did this experience change you? What did you learn from it?
- What effects does it have on your whole life and your environment?
- Are there exceptions where it was not like that? What was different there?
- They say that cult members are always enthusiastic about their group. How would you know if you were in a cult?

About the reaction in the environment

- How does your environment deal with your attitude?
- Which people in your environment benefit from it, and which suffer from it?
- Do you tend to be alone in this or does it also connect you with others? Does it create closeness or distance? Do you get recognition for it, or does it make you more of an outsider? How do you deal with these effects?
- Does XY do you good, or does it rather drag you down? How can you tell that it is good for you, and how can you tell if it does more harm than good?
- How do good friends who have known you for a long time judge your change? Do they think that you are developing positively since you have been dealing with XY? Are they irritated or worried?

- Has your circle of friends changed a lot? Have you reduced contacts with old friends? Why?
- What form of support do you want from me/the family?

About the leading persons

- How do you prevent someone from profiting from your distress?
- One always hears about gurus who abuse their students emotionally, financially or sexually. How do you make sure that your master is not one of them?
- What makes a good mentor or teacher for you? Does he/she fulfill that? Do you feel safe, well cared for, is he/she a person of integrity? Would you act similarly in his/her place? If not, why not? In what case would you not?
- Does the content of the teaching match the actions of the persons in leadership?

About the effects

- Specifically, where do I see XY having a positive impact in your life?
- What should improve in your life in the long run, what might be lost? What might you have to do without if you continue on your path consistently? Is it worth it?
- By when should success be visible?

The miracle question

Miracle question (according to Steve de Shazer [6]): What if a miracle happened and suddenly, while you were asleep, the problem disappeared? When you wake up, it is no longer there. How would you recognize it? What would change as a result? Who in your environment would notice it first?

Be respectful of the answers. You don't need to set clever interventions, give tips, or solve the other person's problems. Asking a good question and listening attentively to the answer without interrupting and without judging the answer is already a precious, rare gift. Listening to understand, not just to have a pause to prepare your own arguments.

Your counterpart notices whether you are genuinely interested in the answers or whether the questions have a purely manipulative character, linked to a specific intention. Before you introduce your own opinion, ask whether the person is interested in your perspective, whether they really can and want to listen.

The author Alexander Eydlin describes in an exciting article in the *ZEIT*, which motives led him to believe in conspiracy myths and which conversations he found helpful in disengaging from them again. He does not find the confrontation with facts purposeful [7]:

> *What helps instead, in my experience, is humility and patience. Whether you tell an honestly interested listener what you think you found out yesterday about covert CIA operations, or you tell it to an ideological opponent who asks rhetorical questions and shakes his head with a smile, there is an enormous difference. The interest of the former is infectious and opens up ways to discover one's own contradictions without judgment. The skepticism of the latter mobilizes defense impulses. Only through the will to understand – not the will to refute – can mental de-escalation be created. Whoever wants to evoke critical thinking must dispense with the habitus of the educator, because education reveals not only the presence of an agenda, i.e. exactly what conspiracy theorists suspect everywhere – but also the same unconditional will to know and to be right, which one criticizes in the counterpart.*

Do not expect that your questions will immediately trigger a change of mind. People change basic attitudes when they have experienced and learned something for themselves that triggers a change. Your questions and your arguments are like seeds that you scatter and that may one day sprout if the conditions are right. Immediately in the conversation, your questions may be brushed aside (*"These are typical questions for the ignorant."*) or answered with great passion for the ideology (*"My guru is the best person who ever lived!"*), but they may develop into slow-burners and have an impact much later. Finding good questions is often harder than finding good arguments. If you don't have a sincere interest in the answers, your counterpart will notice. Then your motivation is to lecture rather than build a bridge of mutual understanding. The most effective tool in the conversation is yourself. Your effectiveness comes from being authentic, tangible, human, and interested in the other person. Also tell about yourself and how your own view of the world came about. What were formative life experiences for you that led to your attitudes today?

If you don't succeed in influencing the views of your counterpart, then at least you will be remembered as a person. In doing so, you change the image of the "opponent" and put black-and-white enemy stereotypes into perspective.

> *In the end, it was not the dogged arguments of those who wanted to prove me wrong that convinced me. But the constant friendships with people who did not share my strange ideas and still saw in me more than a crank. They argued with me, but only*

after they had taken the time to understand my crude ideas. That time, and the respect behind it, and the affection for me as a person were valuable resources that created meaning for me beyond modern myths. The person's behavior was important, not his views. (Alexander Eydlin [7])

Takeaway

A friendly, empathic approach accomplishes more than aggressive, pejorative communication. This is easier to do when one addresses the reasons why a particular belief makes sense to that person, what experience it comes from, and what fears it banishes. There are often well-intentioned motives behind missionary efforts and attempts to win others to that ideology. An interest in the person and an attempt to understand their perspective can accomplish more than trying to fight the ideology alone. The ideology is an expression and fulfillment of a need; if this is understood, alternatives can possibly be brought in.

Addressing the Impact in Everyday Life

"Before enlightenment chop wood, fetch water. After enlightenment chop wood, fetch water." is a saying from Zen Buddhism.

What is crucial is not the one-time spiritual experience, but the transfer to everyday life. Ideals and values must find a concrete expression in everyday life, otherwise they are empty words. Don't be fobbed off with vague statements: *"Since I have been meditating with Guru X, there is much more love in my life."* How does this love come to the fore? In what actions? How would a neighbor recognize this greater extent of love? Who benefits the most, who the least?

You can also stipulate with the proselytizing family member that you would like to wait and observe what positive changes become visible in their life in the coming months/years. If faith is such an excellent help in life, then this must also be visible in the everyday world. With the quote *"By their fruit you will recognize them"* it is also pointed out in the Bible that it is more the results that matter and not so much the intentions. Confront the family member about his or her actions. *"I observe that you speak more pejoratively about others and pigeonhole them more quickly than before. When I criticize you, you seem to get angry and aggressive right away."* is more meaningful than *"You think you people in the group are better than us".*

Are the members of the group in happy relationships? Are they financially secure? Do they work in jobs they enjoy? Are they healthy and vital? Do they spread a positive mood? Are they admired by those around them? Are they role models for people outside the group? Are they actively involved in solving social problems? For example, if a community is particularly committed to world peace: What specifically has been achieved in recent years? What fruit does the commitment bear? How can success be measured? What distinguishes your group from other associations and aid programs?

Since many ideologies claim to offer a superior solution to all of life's questions, the members should also be more successful than average in all areas. Are they?

> Contact with outsiders helped me a lot, for example in school. It was a very, very slow process for me, but I repeatedly noticed that other people were happy, too. That was decisive for me when I realized that happiness doesn't have to be explicitly something that comes only from Jehovah. There are other ways to live. You don't have to be perfect and virtuous. Through outside influences, I realized that it's okay to have your own opinion. (Lisa L.)

Positively Reinforcing Desired Behavior

Prompts like. *"Don't let them manipulate you! They want something from you and are taking advantage of you. Don't be naive and don't give your brains away at the checkroom!"* will most likely trigger resistance in your counterpart. Nobody likes to be given orders. You will probably trigger the impulse in your counterpart to defend their community or themselves. By making a statement like: *"You certainly take good care of yourself and don't let yourself be manipulated so easily. With groups, this is no mean feat. Knowing you, you always retain a modicum of critical reflection,"* formulated as a compliment, the message is conveyed in a way that is more likely to trigger a desire in the other person to live up to the good opinion.

With young people, the world view is not yet set in stone, extreme positions are given a try as part of social learning. Social worker Fabian Reicher's tip when it comes to radicalization:

> I would advise parents to stay emotionally involved with the young person, to stay in touch. There is little point in just attacking the extreme position, especially if everything revolves around this conflict. It is important to look for the exceptions: I don't just criticize what doesn't fit, but I praise when something goes well. Because through negative reinforcement, I still reinforce. The adolescent then thinks, "If I'm nothing else, at least I'm the negative antihero. The more enemies, the more honor."

Focus on the Framework

Ideologies often transfigure the view of the realities of life. In the enthusiasm, facts such as safety, finances, health, couple cohesion, family stability, or child well-being are readily passed over. In a vague way, it is usually assumed that these areas are not important or are automatically improved by the ideology. Especially in fields of esotericism, the reference to plain reality is deliberately abandoned. If you wish the right thing hard enough from the universe, you become rich and healthy. People in the right mindset are automatically successful and happy. Just to doubt it can destroy everything. Then only more seminars help. (*"And maybe you should separate from this critical partner, his negative aura only pulls you down."*) As a result, the fault for failure never lies with the method or the guru himself, but with the person who makes mistakes in the implementation or is "not yet mature enough."

There is usually nothing to be done about the ideology, but some people are willing to consider it on a practical level – but only if they do not feel that it is an attack on the ideology. Create a business plan together, conduct a risk analysis, assist with a labor market research. Invite them to think through the project in a very practical and concrete way, including going through worst-case scenarios. This may meet with resistance from some esoteric people, because for them the very thought of negative developments "attracts" them. In this case I would ask whether this also applies to bridge constructors, air traffic controllers, car mechanics, doctors etc. Do all the problems of our world arise because someone was worried about them? Should these professions from now on not worry about negative effects and only trust firmly in the power of life? Why not? If it is allowed under certain conditions after all, why is your counterpart not allowed to do risk minimization as well?

How much money does the person have available? How much has already been invested, and how long will it take to recoup the cost? What are the job prospects, the general conditions of self-employment, the expected income? How much time can be devoted to the belief system? What can be used to measure success? What could be the effects on the partnership, the family? How can negative effects be counteracted?

Take a Stand, Set Limits

"I don't agree with you, but I'm interested in how you come to that view" is a helpful basic attitude. Easier said than done. This is all the more difficult with topics that affect us emotionally, where we feel personally attacked or where we have a particularly high level of expertise.

Respectful interaction does not mean approving everything and suppressing one's own opinion for the sake of harmony. Sometimes confrontation is sensible and necessary, especially when it comes to inhumane ideologies. Here it is necessary to take a stand. Silence is consent or acquiescence. The more problematic the statement, the more important not to let it stand without comment, even if one does not want to engage in a detailed discussion. Conspiracy myths, for example, are very often anti-Semitic or represent extreme right-wing positions, are slanderous or anti-social. Supporters of these narratives are happy to overlook this. Under the guise of outrage, humanity, respect and decency are often thrown overboard. This can and should be pointed out. Especially in the case of conspiracy myths, it is important to name them as such. In the words of deradicalization expert Fabian Reicher:

> I think it's important to point out what extremism is and to name it. This is a strategy of the so-called new right to normalize racism and other extreme right-wing positions.

***

> In my family WhatsApp group, conspiracy myths and right-wing populist links were increasingly shared. I held back for a long time because I didn't want to disrupt the harmony. I didn't want to be the outsider again, the know-it-all, until it became too much for me. I decided to comment on every post, every link, and post links to fact check sites in response. I networked with people who shared my opinion and who thus backed me up. This has also led to heated arguments with my siblings. However, a nephew of mine contacted me and told me that he admired my stance and that it helped him to speak his mind as well. It is exhausting to go into these arguments, but I feel much more powerful now. I no longer have verbal abuse sold to me as an opinion.

It makes a lot of sense to take a stand yourself, which can be short: *"I don't see it that way." – "That's a conspiracy myth." – "I don't believe that." – "This statement is factually false/anti-Semitic/misogynistic/inhumane/…" – "This is defamation and slander." – "This accusation reduces to simplistic black and white, I see it more complex."*

"I don't believe in astrology, but I can imagine that one is happy about a little tip in life issues."

Trying to understand the other person and build interpersonal bridges does not preclude addressing conflicts and sharing concerns and your own anger. You have no direct influence on a person's beliefs, but you certainly do on the resulting behavior. The entire family does not have to submit to the believer's rules of conduct. Religious freedom also ends where the freedom of other people is curtailed. Some people seek the corset of a very strict regulation of everyday life, which is glossed over and exaggerated by a spiritual ideology. Behind this, however, there can also be obsessive-compulsive disorders, rituals of anxiety defense and despotic behavior, disguised as spiritual obligation.

When conflicts arise in the coexistence of a family or partnership, it is not very useful to swallow anger for a long time. For the ideologically extreme family member, one's own feelings, enthusiasm, sense of mission are often so much in the foreground that the needs of the environment are little perceived or ignored. The setting of clear boundaries is sometimes necessary.

Be aware of your own limits. This also includes accepting that your influence on others is limited and that you will not necessarily achieve more results with more effort.

> I don't go out proselytizing to win. If I succeed in arousing interest in others, it's good, but I don't want to win. I position myself, I assert my position, but I don't want to waste my energy. (Krista Federspiel, journalist)

It may also be that a reduction or even a termination of contact is necessary if you do not succeed in other ways to prevent overbearing behaviour. Not every person can be reached through positive talking strategies. Sometimes it is only after a drastic response, such as blocking messages and excluding them from meetings, that it becomes clear to the person that you mean business. *"The boundary is the actual fruitful place of knowledge."* This phrase by Paul Tillich indicates that insight and change are often only possible when a boundary has been reached and crossed.

> My husband meditated for hours every day. I was often alone with the three children, although he was in the same house. During the remodeling work, he finished his meditation room first, and he was hardly motivated for the rest of the work. He told me that I was too materialistic and that he was walking his spiritual path also for the whole family. He would meditate for the salvation of all of us. My complaints bounced off him. Only when I moved with the children to my parents and he saw that I was serious about a separation, he was suddenly willing to compromise and had more time for the family again. However, I had to strictly insist that the meditation times remain limited, otherwise he would quickly fall back into the old patterns.

> ***

> *When we buy groceries, before each product crosses the threshold of the house, the bar code must be crossed out with a pen. I went along with it at first because it calmed my girlfriend down, but it got more and more extreme with the various regulations to prevent mischief. I then gave her an ultimatum that she had to see a psychiatrist and start psychotherapy or I would break up with her. She was diagnosed with obsessive-compulsive disorder, and with the help of therapy, she soon got much better. Now she is grateful to me for making her do it.*
> ***

> *My son stayed away from my 60th birthday celebration because his spiritual teacher was holding the weekly meditation class online at the time. I tried for a long*

time to be understanding of his spirituality and kept my concerns to myself, but a line was reached. There was a very emotional debate; that's when I told him how much this hurt me and that he talks a lot about divine love but behaves selfishly and heartlessly. We both cried and said some things to each other that we hadn't dared to say before because we both always try to maintain harmony. It was exhausting, but it did us good. He is now turning more consciously to the family again, and the teacher no longer occupies the very first place in his life.

Remain Patient

Changing your mind doesn't happen through radical turnover, but through gradual "nudging" in one direction. (Florian Aigner, science communicator)

As almost all of our interviewees who have experienced a fundamental change in their worldview confirm, attitude changes usually take place over a longer period of time. Sometimes it takes years, and as family members you can make more of an impact with repeated small impulses than with the one big showdown conversation. As a family, you stay connected over a long period of time, sometimes your entire life. Think big, stay in touch, offer other worldviews and values than, for example, those in a cult-like group. What is important to us as a family? That we share hobbies and pursuits, vacations, celebrations and traditions. We are united by a common history. We renovate the house together and are there for each other when someone needs help. Stay patient, make different offers, but also accept when they are rejected. Grass doesn't grow faster if you pull on it. You also need luck and the right offer at the right time.

You have to get rid of the idea that you have immediate communication success. If I succeed in having a good conversation, even if we disagree, a lot has already been achieved. (Martin Puntigam, Science Buster)

***

At the age of 17, my nephew disturbed the family with his radical right-wing views; 10 years later, he himself fought against this ideology as a social worker. When he was 33 he wanted to quit the job to save the world as a shaman and warrior of light, again his parents were horrified. After being very deeply rooted in esotericism for a few years, he has completely withdrawn from it and doesn't want to have anything to do with it anymore. Now he is renovating a farm with his new partner and wants to build a self-sustaining community there. As his uncle, it was easier for me to listen to him than it was for my sister. I often disagreed with him and argued with him a lot, but I always recognised that he was an idealist, a fighter for a better world. I always respected that and liked him, and he knew that. When he had trouble with

his parents, he came to me. We agreed that the world needed to change fundamentally, but disagreed on the methods. Then we went sailing together.
***

As soon as I developed the first doubts, I just listened more, and then I noticed more and more things. It was not one event, but many small ones. (Lisa L.)

Do Not Shame

The people discussed here are often on the defensive, often feel patronized, misunderstood and treated like a child. They do not understand the fear of those around them, see it as a breach of trust when personal information about them is shared with outsiders. They suddenly experience themselves as a problem case in the family, being discussed behind their back.

> I was the same person I'd always been, and suddenly I was treated as if I'd committed a crime, as if I were no longer sane. My husband shared emails from me and my energy healer with family members and also talked to friends about how he feared I was now in a cult. Everyone was talking at me to stop all contact there and then. I felt like I was being put in the pillory stripped naked.

Worrying about a person does not give the right to invade his or her privacy, to obtain hidden personal data and to share it with others. Children and adolescents are an exception to a certain extent. Here, too, however, there is a right to privacy and action should not be taken secretly behind the back of the person concerned.

When a person withdraws from an ideology, leaves a community, possibly admits to mistakes, that is a big step that deserves respect. It is not the time to react with gloating or self-righteousness. As much as possible, help the person save face. Statements like. *"Do you finally see that I was right?"* or. *"I've been telling you that all along!"* are not helpful.

Initially, shame and doubts about one's own ability to judge are often prevalent. Sometimes the entire personal worldview and value system must be reconsidered and the supporting function of ideology and group membership replaced by something new. The more comprehensive and the longer the ideology/community has previously dominated one's life, the greater the loss and struggle with previously made decisions. In problematic communities, there may also have been stressful to traumatic experiences. Many go through a deep personal crisis at this time. Some have hardly any social network left, because breaking away from the community is punished by breaking off contact and the old friendships have been abandoned before. Some have to reorient themselves professionally, some have to rebuild their entire existence. At this point, the family (if it is not part of the system) often proves to be an invaluable resource. It is a safety net, a bridgehead to a new existence, and sometimes the only place where people dare to seek help. It may be that there have been years of estrangement before, that previous slights and hurts on both sides make renewed contact difficult. Nevertheless, many turn to members of the family of origin when in need.

> "You are the average of the five people you spend the most time with," my mentor used to preach. Because I wanted to be special, successful and at a high spiritual level, I greatly reduced contact with my friends and family. They didn't seem to understand me, found only criticism of my mentor and my courses with her, I didn't even want to listen to that anymore. "They pull you into their low frequencies," she said. Only when I realized how superficial and fake this supposedly enlightened woman was, and how much her advice had hurt me, did I seek contact with the family again. I now enjoy how naturally I have been accepted there, that I simply belong and am liked. It feels so good to talk about normal things and experience everyday things together. It helps me to get back in touch with my own needs and to get my feet back on the ground.

> ***

> *My brother was in a commune in South America for 15 years. We had very little contact because the leader of the community forbade it. He lost all contact with his old friends a long time ago. A month ago, he suddenly announced that he could no longer stand it there and that everyone was completely under the thumb of the leader. He is in poor health because he is not allowed to seek medical treatment for his heart condition. His illness is seen as a sign of impurity, he has to stay away from the other members of the community, only the healing treatments of the group are allowed. We immediately collected the money in the family for the ticket home; a cousin made contact with the local consulate so that he could get a passport, the parents gathered the necessary documents. Our sister is taking him in for the first while, another cousin is a nurse and has arranged with a cardiologist at his hospital to see my brother right away and start treatment, even though he doesn't have insurance yet. I'm taking care of the social side and helping him with the applications and all the paperwork. We are so happy to finally have him back with us, and he also says how grateful he is to have family.*

Reflecting on One's Own Contribution

> I think my 33-year-old daughter is in a cult! Until recently, we talked on the phone at least once every day, we spent our vacations together, and she told me everything. Now she wants to go on vacation with friends and doesn't always pick up the phone when I call. She dodges when I ask her questions. There must be a cult behind it. They always try to disrupt contact with the family.

Behind changes in the behavior of a family member, there is not always a cult-like group. Sometimes it is part of developmental phases to break away from the family group for a while; sometimes the family's expectations and orders are inappropriate, or there is transgressive behavior. Changes irritate the environment, even if they are meaningful and necessary. Take a critical look at your own behaviors and family dynamics. Where might you be contributing to your family member's behavior? Are your expectations appropriate for your relative's age? Are you yourself authentic, sincere, fair? Are your expectations reasonable? Could part of the problem also be related to a lack of tolerance and trust on your part? How objectively can you assess the situation? Apply the critical self-reflection you want from the family member to yourself as well. Sometimes the outside perspective of a good friend or therapeutic guidance can help.

Food for Thought

Which people were formative for you and why?

At what stages of your life and through what triggers did you develop or change fundamental attitudes?

Which family members were significant in the development of your own worldview?

Did your family tend to have unity or diversity of views? How were outsiders dealt with? What culture of conversation was cultivated?

Which family member impresses you even though you hold different views and values?

For which people in your current environment can you make a valuable contribution to the development of a critical mind?

7.3   Conflicts in the Partnership

My wife has forbidden the whole family to watch news because they bring negative energies into the house. She searched the bookshelf and removed all the volumes that, according to the master, spread a bad aura. Pictures of the revered master hung everywhere. Then she also started censoring the music I listen to. I felt like I was in prison.

The situation is especially difficult when there are serious differences in world-view within a relationship. Most relationships begin with a basic agreement on important values, views and attitudes. Sometimes a partner develops in a different direction, discovers a religion for himself or breaks away from it, changes his political attitude or becomes more radical in his views. This quickly leads to ongoing trench warfare, where people try to prove the other person wrong by all means. Some of these discussions are exciting, harmless and add spice to the relationship. But when it comes to a topic where the effects are more problematic or other people are involved, the blood pressure rises. Is the daughter's neurodermatitis treated by an alternative practitioner or with cortisone? Are the children vaccinated or not? Does the vacation have to be postponed because Medium Esmeralda predicts a plane crash? Does the partner also have to attend the group meetings because otherwise the master sees no future for the relationship?

The wacky quirk that was charming at the beginning of the relationship, the commitment to movement XY that was admired at first, can lead to increasing irritation over time. Time, money, energy are used by the partner for something for which one has less and less understanding. Sometimes a divergence of views only arises in the course of the relationship, for example, when one of the partners turns to a spiritual movement, changes strongly in his (social) political views or becomes increasingly interested in conspiracy myths.

One client put it this way:

We liked to discuss things at the beginning of our relationship, but we agreed on important issues. Now I sometimes think to myself that I don't even know this man. Recently, he seriously told me that the most important politicians are all alien lizard creatures disguised to take over the Earth. How can I still respect him when he holds such views? I feel embarrassed when he talks about it among our friends.

When the fundamental ideological basis in a relationship drifts apart, it creates fast-growing gaps that are difficult to bridge.

Anticipate that you will not be able to change your partner. If you assume that the different belief positions are constant, is there still enough connection? How can living together still work?

Relationship Tip

When there are differing views on important issues, two things are especially important:

1. **Mutual tolerance:** no constant trench warfare and attempts at missionary work. It must be possible for **both** to be able to respect the other person, even if you have different attitudes. You can reject the attitude, but you must keep your appreciation for the person. To clarify, it is helpful to go to

the meta-level of the relationship and discuss how you feel about the other person holding that position: *"We have different points of view, how do we deal with that? What does it trigger in you that I don't share your view? How do I feel about that?"* The issue should not consume the majority of resources in the relationship; it should not be all about this disagreement all the time. Sometimes this disagreement masks other couple conflicts, and sometimes it serves as a rationale or final push to end a relationship that is already drifting apart.

2. **Connecting:** Work consciously to see that there are other areas that connect you as a couple, where there are common interests and shared views. Consciously notice what is beautiful, beneficial and strengthening in the relationship, what you appreciate in the other person. The different worldviews (if they trigger strong negative emotions) create a repulsion reaction, like magnets with the same polarity. You need good common ground and good everyday experiences that connect and strengthen you as a couple to counteract this.

I spent hours on the computer watching conspiracy theory videos and blogs. I was completely immersed in that world. It didn't do me any good at all. The people posting there are so full of fear and hate, the whole world seems to be on the brink. It was like a drug, I couldn't get away from it. Every day the first thing I did was read up on what new signs were proving the great takeover of the world by the dark cabal. It was a euphoric feeling to be among the few "awakened" ones. At the same time I felt more and more restless and empty and lost the ground under my feet. Then my life partner opened up to me that he could no longer live with me like this. He cried and said that he felt helpless because he saw that I was not well and that he could not reach me anymore. He said he didn't recognize the woman he fell in love with and that he would have to end the relationship if I wasn't willing to work with him on it. This was a big shock to me. I knew he was unhappy, but not how much it was bothering him, and that I was about to lose him. We then agreed that as a first measure I would do a complete online withdrawal from the relevant sites for three weeks and we would take time for ourselves and go out into nature a lot and to the mountains, which was always our favorite hobby together. At first, that didn't work. If I wanted to see my sister's Facebook messages, I couldn't avoid those of the other groups either. I also noticed how often I reached for my cell phone because I wanted to distract myself, was bored, or was afraid of missing something. Then I read an article about a digital detox challenge. Over the course of 30 days, the smartphone is used less and less [8]. My partner agreed to do it with me. He found it even harder than I did. Suddenly I was no longer the "problem case" in the relationship, but we fought together against our bad habits. This bonded us a lot, we suffered together, had fun together and had to engage with each other a lot more again. After the 30 days, I radically reduced all social media activity. I deleted most pages and created new accounts in some cases. I couldn't say I've renounced conspiracy theories, but I know they don't do me any good. I don't want to deal with it and avoid even

*thinking about it. When the topic comes up on the news, I tune out. Right now
that helps me the most, and it has saved my relationship.*

If there are children together, this conflict often intensifies. For example, if a
religion is very important to one parent and the other parent strictly rejects
this commitment to faith, a conflict usually erupts over the manner and intensity in which this faith should be taught to the children.

A practical example:

*Mrs. X's husband has joined Jehovah's Witnesses after a few years of relationship.
Mrs. X rejects the community and does not want their two common children to
attend meetings and children's Bible courses. For Mr. X, however, it is very important that he teaches his children these values and contents. Otherwise, in his view,
he would be making a serious mistake as a father and exposing his children to a
dangerous future without the protection of faith. In some areas, such as celebrating birthdays and Christmas, the couple quickly finds compromises; in others, constant discussions ensue: Are the children allowed to read Harry Potter books? Are
posters of music bands in the children's rooms problematic? Can Mr. X take the
children with him when he makes house calls as a missionary? Mrs. X does not
want him to tell the children about sin, God's punishment and the temptations of
the devil. It annoys him that she lets the children watch or read (from his point of
view) harmful films and books.*

More on this in the next chapter.

Takeaway

If a change in views does not seem possible, then much is already gained if
friend-foe thinking can be countered. Respect for other opinions can only be
demanded if it is also exemplified oneself.

Despite all understanding and empathy, it remains important to recognize
and maintain one's own boundaries. Misanthropic, radicalizing ideologies should
not be legitimized and normalized through silence. Protecting and delimiting
oneself and, in the worst case, ending a contact remains an option. Changes in
worldview often take place over many years; the family is an important resource,
especially from the onset of doubts and after a change.

References

1. https://www.mimikama.at
2. Petzold H, Orth I (1994) Kreative Persönlichkeitsdiagnostik durch mediengestützte Techniken in der Integrativen Therapie und Beratung. In: Petzold H (Hrsg) Integrative Therapie. Zeitschrift für vergleichende Psychotherapie und Methodenintegration, Bd 20. Junfermann, Paderborn, S 312–391

3. Neuberger S (2018) Menschen auf der Suche: Beratung und Psychotherapie im Umfeld von sogenannten Sekten und weltanschaulichen Gemeinschaften vor dem Hintergrund systemischen Denkens. Facultas Universitätsverlag, Wien, p 90

4. Schleichert H (2012) Wie man mit Fundamentalisten diskutiert, ohne den Verstand zu verlieren: Anleitung zum subversiven Danken, 7. Aufl. Beck, München S 150–151

5. Hain P (2009) Humor und Hypnotherapie. In: Revenstorf D, Peter B (eds) Hypnose in Psychotherapie, Psychosomatik und Medizin. Springer, Heidelberg, pp 162–166

6. de Shazer S (2006) Der Dreh: Überraschende Wendungen und Lösungen in der Kurzzeittherapie. Carl-Auer, Heidelberg

7. Ich sah das Schlachtfeld von Alexander Eydlin. https://www.zeit.de/kultur/2020-09/verschwoerungstheorien-anhaenger-erfahrung-umgang-vorurteile-coronavirus. Accessed on: 21. Febr. 2021

8. https://www.forbes.com/sites/nextavenue/2017/01/04/try-the-30-day-digital-detox-challenge/. Accessed on: 1. Mai 2020

8

Children and Adolescents

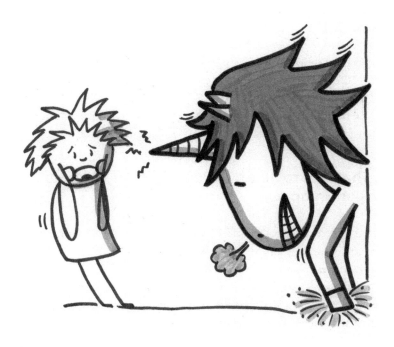

H. G. Hümmler, U. Schiesser, *Fact and Prejudice*,
https://doi.org/10.1007/978-3-662-66032-4_8

8.1   Problem Areas

I am an elementary school teacher. A 7-year-old girl in my class told me enthusiastically that she and her mother are training to be healers. There she learns to put her hands on people's heads, and then the energy of the universe comes and heals people. I asked the child's mother about this and she confirmed that she takes her daughter to training groups of an esoteric venture, and that this was expressly desired by the organization. Children could attend for free up to the age of 15. They were especially good healers because they had a much better vibration than adults and therefore worked especially well as a spiritual channel [1].

***

My daughter is five years old. She had heart surgery when she was a baby, and she has to have annual checkups. My ex-girlfriend canceled the appointment this year. She stated at the hospital that she will go to another clinic. In truth, she is going to a healer who assured her that he would cure her daughter and that already the first surgery had been unnecessary. My ex has sole custody, I don't even get to see the medical records.

Children and adolescents are primarily affected in two areas[1]:

1. As a target group of various offers,
2. As those directly affected, who grow up in an environment that is shaped by their parents' religious, political, or ideological attitudes.

Offers That Aim to Reach Children and Adolescents as a Target Group

There are always associations and individuals who, without sound pedagogical evidence and training, place their, often ideological, offers at schools and childcare facilities. Sometimes the origin of the offer is not communicated, e.g. in the case of "Youth for Human Rights" and "Foundation for a Drug-Free World," which are initiated by Scientology members. In addition to the commitment to socially recognized issues (e.g., peace), one's own community and ideology are often promoted inconspicuously. One example of this is "Operation Christmas Child," a popular and widespread project that presents disadvantaged children with toys and school supplies packed in a shoebox at Christmas. Little known is that this project originates from "Samaritan's

---

[1] Parts of the text with amendments already published in the Activity Report of the Federal Agency for Sectarian Issues 2019: https://www.parlament.gv.at/PAKT/VHG/XXVII/III/III_00175/index.shtml accessed on 09.02.2021.

Purse," an evangelical association that also sees missionizing as an important goal of the distribution campaign. Communities such as Scientology send unsolicited books and CDs/DVDs of their movement to schools as donations for school libraries or as learning materials for subjects such as addiction education, ethics or sex education.

In our kindergarten, we were invited to an information event. The topic was how to recognize and promote the talents and abilities of the next generation. The speaker presented a program that was supposedly scientifically proven. With the help of the date and time of birth, a chart would be created for each child, which could be used to identify talents and limitations. I was immediately skeptical and even during the lecture I read critical reports on the Internet on my smartphone. However, my objections bounced off the lecturer, and I was shocked at how many of the parents hung on his every word and enthusiastically embraced his parenting instructions.

Dubious products such as food supplements, "energized" remedies, talismans, various treatments and programs are offered to parents for ADHD, autism, allergies, dyslexia, developmental delays and every conceivable ailment. These range from harmless remedies to life-threatening products such as MMS (Miracle Mineral Supplement), a chlorine dioxide solution that has for example been administered as an enema to autistic children in the hope that they would be cured in this way. Using equipment and methods that do not stand up to scientific scrutiny, diagnoses are made (often by medical laymen) and treatments recommended. For example, kinesiological muscle tests are used to determine alleged allergies in children, who are then usually told to avoid white flour, sugar, dairy products and the like for a long period of time, which can be a great burden and harmful to a child's health. Often parents are advised not to have their children vaccinated; sometimes urgently needed medical treatments are not carried out because the medical diagnosis is doubted or an alternative treatment concept is promoted. Accompanying evidence based medical care, these treatments and products can be quite harmless or even helpful. In the case of chronic illnesses of children and adolescents such as diabetes, cystic fibrosis, epilepsy or acute illnesses such as cancer and infections, there can be a life-threatening danger if parents rely exclusively on spiritual or alternative healing methods.

The conflict came when our child was born and I experimented with homeopathic remedies, which did not work at all. My partner said: "You are not objective, let the pediatrician treat it." (Thomas F., pediatrician)

Children as Direct Victims

The development of children and adolescents in safety and freedom can be endangered by extreme religious or ideological beliefs of parents. That may be because they grow up in great fear, on the one hand, of a punishing God who would constantly watch the child, record his offenses in a "sin register" and punish disobedience, and on the other hand, of a demonic influence that would always try to seduce the child into undesirable behavior. Also when children are taught that they are growing up in a dangerous and endangered world, constantly threatened by overpowering negative forces. Even the instruction that one must always cherish only positive thoughts and must always conform to a certain canon of rules can cause great stress. A spiritual perfectionism is sometimes expected that is almost impossible to fulfill, and thus children and young people are left with the constant feeling of failing, of sinning, of not being good enough, or of endangering others by their behavior. These "offenses" sometimes include normal feelings and impulses such as anger, jealousy, resentment, and sexual desire. One's own impact on the world may be overestimated (*"Because I had this negative thought, so many people died in the earthquake in Haiti."*), but also underestimated (*"My needs don't matter as long as the community is doing well" "I am nothing without my faith."*). It is particularly problematic when religious writings recommend educational methods that are out of date, for example, when beating children is not only recommended as a legitimate instrument of correction, but even required of parents as a "proof of love" (*"Those who spare the rod hate their children, but those who love them are diligent to discipline them."* [2]).

> *Since the children were taught that the parents were acting on a divine educational mandate, there was always the threat that disobedience and rebellion against the parents would also result in God's punishment, up to and including the loss of salvation. My friends of the same age and I developed a behavior towards all adults that was strongly characterized by conformity and submissiveness* [3]. (Anna, Report of a Dropout)

Social contact outside the community is sometimes made difficult, attendance at school events is forbidden, and books, movies, and media that children are allowed to consume are heavily regulated and controlled. Time-consuming religious obligations often leave children and adolescents little time to meet with peers and develop alternative interests; they experience themselves as outsiders, strangers and insecure in the social environment outside their own community.

In kindergarten I often heard, "Now Sarah has to go out of the room, we're celebrating a birthday now." Or Christmas, Easter, St. Nicholas. And then I stood in the hallway while the others sang and ate cake. For me, there has never been a birthday celebration. I tried to imagine everyone in the group being punished by Jehovah, but I didn't really want that either, they were my friends. At school I was "the Jehovah's Witness kid" and an outsider. The mother of a classmate demanded that her daughter would not sit next to me in the bench, because she was afraid that I would proselytize her daughter, as if I were contagious.

Excessive religious or ideological commitment on the part of parents can also lead to neglect of children. Children's needs become secondary to the demands of the community, and some communities even require members to "disengage" from ties, to set aside relationships and responsibilities in favor of spirituality. Time-consuming faith obligations and practices can greatly dominate and restrict family life.

Faith communities often develop their own ideas, about the origins of illnesses, which can stand in the way of medical treatment; mental illnesses in particular often do not receive adequate diagnosis and treatment.

Another area of conflict arises when parents take different positions, when one parent rejects the spiritual commitment or ideological orientation of the other parent and sees this as a threat to the children they share. Such conflicts often lead to custody proceedings in court and are conducted with high emotionality. The children find themselves in an enormous conflict of loyalties, not only between the parents, but also between two different religious values, basic attitudes and views of the world.

My ex-boyfriend refuses to recognize the legitimacy of the state and adheres to various conspiracy myths. He conveys to our mutual 13-year-old son that school is not important because the system will soon collapse anyway. He seems to move more and more in a right-wing extremist environment. Recently he took our son to a survival training in the forest. There were weapons drills to defend against the supposedly imminent "Great Replacement". My son wants to please his father and thinks the militant behavior of the others is cool. I find all this disgusting and do not want my son to come into contact with this ideology. With my ex-boyfriend, any discussion about it is pointless.

Social isolation, ideological compartmentalization and dependence on the religious community hinder the development of a self-reliant personality that can move in our society in a self-determined manner, seize professional and educational opportunities and develop in freedom. The right to freely practice one's religion and the rights of parents to teach their children their own values and world views are important fundamental rights of a democracy. However, they must not be at the expense of the rights of children and adolescents: the right to develop one's personality, the protection of human dignity, the right to life and physical integrity. Religious freedom must not come at the expense of children's rights [4].

> **Takeaway**
>
> The rights of children as set forth in the UN Convention on the Rights of the Child take precedence over the rights of parents to teach religious or political beliefs. The right to health, freedom of expression, non-violent upbringing and education must not be hindered by the ideology of parents. As a society, we share responsibility for ensuring that children and adolescents can participate in a diverse, liberal democracy, seize professional and educational opportunities, and develop into independent personalities.

My divorced wife wants to travel to Croatia with our 15-year-old daughter for a yoga week. At first I thought this was a good idea. My daughter is very sensitive, rather shy, suffers from test anxiety and quickly takes everything to heart. I thought yoga and meditation could help her relax better when she is stressed. However, upon further inquiry, it turned out that they are going to a guru that my ex-wife worships. They will live in his shared apartment and book an intensive week of his self-developed esoteric technique together with his disciples. Then on the Internet I found negative reports about him, that he practices free sexuality with his disciples and works with some kind of sexual magic. I definitely don't want my daughter to go there. Who knows what they do there and if she can say no in that situation. My ex thinks it's none of my business; and my daughter has been looking forward to vacationing by the sea and doesn't want to get into any stress with her mother either.

8.2   Tips for Parents in Custody Conflicts

- A parent's membership in a religious/spiritual group, an anti-state movement, or sympathizing with an otherwise problematic ideology is not in itself a sufficient criterion for endangering the child's welfare [5], even if it is a community about which there has already been much critical reporting. There must be concrete evidence of this endangerment; it does not matter whether the endangerment is physical, mental or emotional.
- Do not put children in conflicts of loyalty! Do not make fun of the spirituality and worldview of the other parent in front of your child. Disparaging

remarks and loudly expressed horror at his or her activities could cause your child not to tell you anything in the future ("*What esoteric crap has your mother bought again. Those angel drops are total bullshit, you're not taking them!*"). Any conflict between parents causes stress for children, and they sometimes avoid it by not bringing up problematic issues in the first place.

- This doesn't mean that you can't take a stand and represent different positions. But do so in a way that relates to factual aspects and does not slip into emotional devaluation: "*Your mother believes that angels exist and that you can put the magical power of these angels into drops of water. I do not believe that angels exist. And if they do, I don't believe their powers are in this water. I think this is something that people wish for. We'd all like to be able to do magic.*"

- Try to see in the other parent first and foremost the father/mother of your child and not your ex-partner. You may be angry because he/she behaved badly, hurt you, lied to you and cheated on you. There were reasons why the relationship failed. Still, the person can be a good father/mother for the child you have together. Try to stay on the parenting level and not keep bringing in old hurts and conflicts from the couple level. This is much easier said than done, but if you yourself want to be a good father/mother to your child, then this is an essential contribution. When a child says, "*I don't want to go to daddy/mommy,*" this can also be an expression of the conflict of loyalty. Can I go to my dad's/mom's house, or will you be angry with me? Can I have a good time there, too? A statement such as: "*I want you to go to your dad's/mom's house, and I want you to be happy and have fun there,*" can relieve a child of this burden. If complaints persist, the cause must of course be investigated.

- Encourage independent thinking, critical questioning and a good discussion culture at an early age. Support the development of your child's own point of view: "*What do you think? What's your opinion?*" Convey education, liberal and democratic values, and the fascination of science, even in areas other than the ideological conflict field:

  - Visit museums, possibly with a guided tour for children. Many museums also offer children's birthday parties with an appropriate program.
  - Long Night of Science [6], of Research [7], of Museums, of Culture
  - Children's University: Many universities and colleges offer events that aim to teach science to children [8]. For example, the Vienna Children's University [9] opens the doors of Vienna's universities for 2 weeks in the

summer for children aged 7–12. They meet scientists in lectures and finish their studies with a graduation ceremony.

- Participate in a research project together: Citizen Science [10].
- Cabaret programs such as the Science Busters, Vince Ebert
- Science Slams [11].
- Children's books, picture books, comics that convey knowledge or deal with inclusion, tolerance, and diversity of lifestyles (e.g., "Alles Familie" by Alexandra Maxeiner).
- Science-promoting television productions: Sendung mit der Maus, Willi will's wissen, Löwenzahn, Was ist was, Wissen macht Ah!, Wow – die Entdeckerzone, …
- Online: www.haus-der-kleinen-forscher.de, Vienna Museum of Technology [12], IST Austria [13], Young Science [14], ScienceLab [15].
- YouTube: "MrWissen2go", "MaiLab", "MEGA", "Wild Mics – Ferngespräch", "Quarks", "Kurzgesagt – In a Nutshell", "It's okay to be smart", "Jubilee" "Vsauce", "Checker Welt"

- It's not enough to just position yourself as the antithesis. What are your own values and attitudes, what is your view of the world? Do you find the state-denying attitude of your ex-partner impossible? What are your political attitudes? What are important democratic values that you want to convey? It takes effort to address these issues and then to translate the answers into concrete action. Fanatics don't shy away from this and are often more eloquent and well versed due to their intensive engagement with their views. As a result, they convey a certainty that is attractive to some.
- *"There is no point in educating children, they imitate everything we do anyway."* This sentence is attributed to Karl Valentin and sums up an important piece of wisdom: your practical example has a more formative effect than lectures. Parents' attitudes are transmitted to their children quite automatically, even if the subject is not addressed directly. When parents agree and frame the environment as a closed bubble, children have no choice but to perceive their parents' view as "the reality." It is only in confrontation with other views – often this happens through friends or at school – that important differentiation emerges. The picture of the world becomes more complex and multifaceted. Diversity of opinion and uncertainties, coincidence and injustice must now be integrated. One parent represents a problematic belief system? All the more important that the other parent, as well as grandparents, uncles and aunts, and other caregivers, are available as anchors for other worldviews. Just knowing *"There's*

another way to look at this" counteracts tunnel vision and helps children and teenagers develop their own positions.

- In order for you to have the opportunity to communicate your worldview at all, it is crucial that the contact with your child does not break off. This often means compromising with the second parent, especially if residency and custody are not equally divided. Pick your battles! If the other parent insists that the child get emergency drops (Bach Flower Remedies) when he or she bumps his or her knee, then a conflict of principle is usually not worth it. If emergency drops are the only intervention allowed even for serious injuries, then confrontation is important.
- Be especially careful to have a say in medical decisions. In many areas of esotericism, there is a hostile attitude toward evidence-based medicine. Various pseudo-diagnosis procedures are offered and ineffective, sometimes even highly dangerous treatment methods are promoted. Vaccinations are often rejected, necessary treatments are not allowed. Act as an advocate for the interests of the child and do not shy away from conflict here. The well-being of the child trumps freedom of belief.
- Be patient and think long term. Parenting is a marathon, not a sprint. You remain a significant factor throughout your child's life. Even after phases of estrangement, rapprochement and a good parent-child relationship can occur again. Especially during puberty or early adulthood, these are sometimes part of the developmental process. If one parent lives an ideology radically, this parent will often try to push the other parent completely out of the child's life. The belief construct is often used as a weapon: "*You have a very negative aura when you come back from visits to your mother. Until that dissipates, you can't play with the other kids, they'll get infected.*"
- Stay persistent, and keep making offers of contact!

8.3 Informing Authorities

Deciding whether to involve authorities in conflict issues is not easy. There is a justifiable fear that the conflict will then escalate even further. In the worst case, the official in charge may sympathize with the ideology and show solidarity with the fanatic parent. However, it is also possible that extreme excesses of the ideology are kept in check by involving the child protective services. The stronger you fear a threat to the child's well-being, the more important this step is. It may be possible to first seek anonymous advice from the authority as to how the situation is assessed there and what steps they advise you to take. In Austria, a request can also be made to the Children's and Youth

Advocates's Office (Kinder- und Jugendanwaltschaft) to clarify this decision [16]. The child or adolescent him/herself can also contact one of these offices directly. It is also possible for both parents to jointly make use of a mediation session at a family center. In Austria, conflict support and family counseling are offered by various agencies. In Germany, the youth welfare offices, and often schools or daycare centers as well, can provide contact to appropriate counseling centers. The neutral view from the outside can de-escalate and bring the interests of the child to the fore. Do not be afraid of child protection agencies; they serve to support families and represent the interests of children and adolescents [17].

If you, as neighbors, relatives, people close to the child, notice a problematic development, involving the authorities is an important option. This can also be done anonymously; however, a personal submission is better, as follow-up questions are possible here and details can be clarified. Especially if both parents radically share the same ideology, we as an environment are obliged [18] to act and not look the other way. In Austria, a report can also be made via an online form [19].

Takeaway

If there is disagreement among parents about the religious and ethical upbringing of children, the child should not be swept up in a conflict of loyalties. Both parents should (as far as possible) accept each other's position and communicate their own worldview independently. Children can learn that there are many different religions and points of view. An independent formation of opinion and view of the world should be encouraged at an early age. Family members can contribute aspects that are neglected in the parental home. If religious or ideological guidelines endanger the well-being of the child, the environment is obligated to intervene.

8.4   Tips for Social and Educational Workers

- Often it is the particularly quiet, well-behaved children whose needs are overlooked. Often, religious communities particularly enforce obedience and respect for the community's authorities. Under these conditions, suffering manifests itself less as rebellion and more as mental or psychosomatic illness or eating disorder.
- Children and adolescents are sometimes urged to keep religious affiliation secret out of concern for discrimination and prejudice. Adolescents sometimes lead a double life. They change clothes between home and school, for

example, and act very differently with their peers than they do in the religious community. They often have the experience of becoming outsiders in the classroom because of the values and rituals of the group.

- Problematic ideological communities always have the dogma of being an elite and thus superior to others. The outsider position is positively reinterpreted by devaluing non-members. This often results in an arrogant attitude that rejects the values, rules and instructions of "others of a different faith" and does not accept them as valid for the members. This also increases the gap between a child from this community and the environment. The Vienna Children's and Youth Advocate's Office reports, *"And some are so caught up in feelings of fear, shame and guilt that even when someone tries to help them, they experience this offer of help as a threat because they have completely lost the ability to perceive their own feelings. This is something that happens to children who grow up in radical religious groups"* [20].

As early as elementary school age, we children were prepared to bravely endure "defamation for the sake of our faith" like martyrs. We should see this as an award for our virtue and rejoice in it. Negative feedback from my social environment regarding my religious ideology thus bounced off me like off a wall [3]. (Anna, Report of a Dropout)

- Does the intense religious commitment still leave parents enough time to devote to their children? How much time does a child spend in meditation, Bible circles, training, rituals, and community gatherings? How much time is left for their own free development? Are the assignments appropriate for children and their age? Do they meet modern pedagogical standards?
- **Warning signals:** the child is banned from activities, books, and movies that are common in the age group. The child is not allowed to participate in some classroom activities for religious reasons. Educational material is rejected that covers topics such as sex education, equality, LGBTIQ[2]-rights, evolution, the values of the liberal, diverse society. Parents try to limit contact with peers; extreme political and religious worldviews are prevalent in the child's environment. The values conveyed there either contradict democratic society or fundamentally reject state frameworks.

Scientific literature, e.g. on the theory of evolution, psychological literature and many works of children's literature (e.g. Harry Potter, The Little Ghost, ...) were judged to be diabolical, demonic or occult and should not be read. Children were also kept

---

[2] LGBTIQ: Abbreviation for Lesbian, Gay, Bisexual, Transgender, Intersexual, Queer.

away from music genres such as rock, pop, metal, etc. Many popular movies, television shows, and youth magazines (Sabrina, Bravo, etc.) were also frowned upon as devilish. Harmless school teaching aids such as yoga exercises or coloring mandalas were refused because of their alleged "occult" reference. Instead, we were given Christian children's literature, movies, and music, and were expected to study creationism. My cultural horizon was thus limited, and I was unable to have a say in many of the topics that were important to my classmates [3]. (Anna, Report of a Dropout)

- When talking to teachers or social workers, parents often succeed in downplaying ideological differences. Most are aware in advance of critical points of friction with the basic values of modern, liberal society. Some communities provide concrete help on how to respond to questions and accusations, or are quick to threaten legal action in the event of criticism. The right to free exercise of religion is often cited, and criticism or even inquiry is dismissed as discrimination.
- Children and young people who do not identify with the values of these groups often feel lonely and disconnected. Especially when parents engage only within the ideological bubble, school and vocational training represent an important bridge to the big wide world. This makes the role of teachers and kindergarten teachers, who can become a confidant, all the more important. The competence center "Right-wing Extremism and the Family" [21] states: *"Professionals should ensure that children experience a culture of behavioral alternatives, equality and appreciative treatment of perceived differences and can learn central democratic principles such as having a say, participating, formulating their own opinion and accepting other opinions"* [22].
- Education generally represents an important factor in breaking free financially and ideologically from a cult-like group. It does not make one immune, but less susceptible to conspiracy myths and pseudoscientific claims.

In school, people are encouraged to think for themselves and to question things critically so that they can understand them better. But in assembly, that is considered intellectually weak, and that has never made sense to me. If it is not welcome to question a teaching and just use your own mind, it looks to me as if the framework of faith taught has gaps and cannot withstand questions. This made me very suspicious and led me to ask critical questions, which was an important point in my liberation process. (Lisa L.)

***

We make a big mistake, a really big mistake, when we think that a successful educational intervention means "winning" the discussion. In fact, I think it's a big mistake when youth facilities immediately ban people for making certain statements. It is important to take a stand against inhumane statements, but it is usually not very effective to immediately start arguing. As an adult, I can argue down a 15-year-old as much as I want. And what he learns is that the strongest wins the discussion. That's how I indirectly teach authoritarianism. The stronger one is right. He may be more likely to change his position if I treat him appreciatively. In many situations it is pedagogically more effective to let opinions stand side by side and to make sure that the setting in which the discussions take place is a democratically organized framework. I will not win this with sanctions; my pedagogical goal is that the young people I work with develop an "inner autonomy," that is, thinking and acting from their own values. Political education is not successful if the young person says and thinks exactly what I think and say. That contradicts the whole concept. They should develop their own positions and neither believe me nor any propagandists everything! (Fabian Reicher, social worker)

- Take signals seriously: What stands out that does not correspond to behavior that is normal for the age group? Ask what meaning it has.
- Take concerns of a second parent (or grandparents, neighbors, etc.) about a religion and worldview seriously, e.g. in custody proceedings.
- Establish rapport, ask open (follow-up) questions, do not devalue the religious group in front of the child, this creates loyalty conflicts.
- Possible questions that can be asked:

  - What are the different religions in your family? Which one do you have?
  - What is important in that religion? What are the tenets of the faith? Where does this show up in everyday life?
  - What is right and wrong behavior?
  - What happens when someone behaves wrongly?
  - What are the rules, rituals, festivals? What are sacred places, objects, dates, concepts?
  - Who is in charge, who has authority? How does one get it?
  - Do women have the same rights and responsibilities as men?
  - Is it okay to criticize? Who does it most often? What happens then?
  - What do you agree on, where do you disagree?
  - Is it okay to make fun of content or the community? Is humor allowed?
  - What happens if you don't pray, don't attend the service? Are there penalties?
  - How much time do you spend each day/weekend on your religion? Are there compulsory appointments such as religious education classes, bible

study groups, common events? Is this amount of time okay for you? What would you change if you could?

- When you are sick, are there specific rules in your religion? How are sick people supported? Do they also go to the doctor, or use predominantly prayer to help them get well? Is sickness a sign of sin, a sign that you have done something wrong?
- Is it your job to recruit people to your faith? In what way? How do you feel about it?
- Are there people in your family who are not believers? How do you deal with them? Do you have contact with them? Do they face punishment?
- What do you think of people who don't have your faith?
- Do you have friends who are not of your religion?
- If you fall in love with someone who does not belong to your religious community, is that a problem? What happens then? Are there several couples in your community who have different faiths?
- What would happen if you joined another religion? What would be the reaction? Who would be most opposed to it, who would be most happy about it? Would you be treated differently? Are there people with whom you would no longer be able to have contact?

These questions refer primarily to a religiously influenced parental home. Accordingly adapted, they are also to be applied to parents with strongly esoteric ideas or to parents who adhere to conspiracy myths, who reject the state, whose worldview and political extremism lead to isolation and alienation of the children.

> With children, I wouldn't start to argue, but show empathy: "It's perfectly fine that you are a Jehovah's Witness, we accept that. If you need anything or have any questions, about anything, feel free to come to me." Just offer and keep emphasizing, "You're safe here, this is a Safe Space. You can say whatever you want here too, you don't have to worry about us telling your parents or elders." There is no such thing as a Safe Space at the Witnesses. There's a snitch system there, anybody can snitch on you, you have to tiptoe all the time. And making that clear to a kid, "You can say whatever you want here, it's not leaving this room," that would have helped me a lot at the time. (Lisa L.)

- If the child/adolescent belongs to the LGBTIQ spectrum, that is, is homo- bi- or intersexual or identifies as transgender or nonbinary, it is important to pay special attention to whether this leads to problems with the community and whether coming out there is even possible. Is there a stigma associated with sexual orientation and gender identity? Is it interpreted as a sin, a form of obsession, a blemish? Fundamental religious communities often include homophobic and transphobic teachings. Growing up in this environment can be an additional complication to building a confident identity and developing a positive approach to one's sexuality.

- In general, sexuality and desire are often taboo and almost forbidden as "dirty." This often applies to any form of sexuality that takes place outside of marriage, including masturbation. Young people are then faced with the dilemma of either violating religious commandments and incurring guilt or having to suppress all sexual desire (even in thought). This puts them in stark contrast to their peer group outside the community, and it also influences their first relationships, sometimes resulting in early marriages.

- Beware of preconceptions about communities, whether positive or negative! Religious communities are complex and have many facets. For example, do not make assumptions about free churches from your own experiences with the Catholic Church. Don't assume you understand a yoga guru group because you've taken a yoga class. Don't judge a community solely on its neat self-promotion, but also don't judge it solely on critical dropout reports. The experience in a cult-like community often shows certain typical characteristics, but is also individual like a fingerprint. Every case is an individual case.

The mere fact that parents belong to a (new) religious group should not necessarily lead to the conclusion that they are unsuitable to raise their children. (…) And at the same time, the appeal to freedom of faith on the part of the parents must not lead to too high a tolerance threshold with regard to the best interests of the child. (Brochure "Freedom of Faith versus the Welfare of the Child" by Sekten-Info NRW) [23].

- Religion is not a taboo. Treat this area as you would other burdensome or relieving factors in psychology and social work.

> **Takeaway**
>
> If you work professionally or as a volunteer with children and young people, be careful not to overlook the silent and conformist. Religion, in both positive and negative ways, can be a powerful impact factor that should not be ignored. Address the issue, provide a safe place to reflect on it. The best interests of the child take precedence over the right of parents to teach their faith.

Food for Thought

What influence did your parents' or early environment's religion have on you?

Were there positive and negative effects on your self-worth, sense of safety and security, self-efficacy, connectedness and belonging?

How has your spiritual map changed over the course of your life?

What would you want to pass on to a child today?

Are there children and youth in your environment who are exposed to destructive beliefs? Do you intervene? Why yes, why no? In what ways could you be supportive?

Could it be that you yourself are imparting incriminating worldviews with the best of intentions?

If you work with children and youth yourself: How much attention have you paid to the topic of faith so far? What experiences and prejudices influence your views? Do you act particularly cautiously, particularly brashly as a result?

References

1. Angebot auf der Homepage von Access Consciousness https://www.accessconsciousness.com/de/micrositesfolder/accessbars/youth/access-kids-2020/. Accessed on: 09.Febr.2021
2. Proverbs 13:24
3. Erfahrungsbericht einer Aussteigerin, veröffentlicht auf der Homepage der Kinder- und Jugendanwaltschaft Wien. https://kja.at/site/files/2020/04/EVZ-Aussteigerbericht-Anonym.pdf. Accessed on: 9. Febr. 2021
4. Nachzulesen in der Kinderrechtskonvention der Vereinten Nationen. https://unicef.at/fileadmin/media/Kinderrechte/crcger.pdf. Accessed on: 9. Febr. 2021
5. Kriterien für eine Gefährdung des Kindeswohls (Österreich). https://www.jusline.at/gesetz/abgb/paragraf/138. Accessed on: 9. Febr. 2021
6. https://www.langenachtderwissenschaften.de. Accessed on: 6. Febr. 2021
7. https://www.langenachtderforschung.at. Accessed on: 6. Febr. 2021
8. Eintrag zu „Kinderuniversität" in Wikipedia. https://de.wikipedia.org/wiki/Kinderuniversität. Accessed on: 9. Febr. 2021
9. https://kinderuni.at
10. https://www.citizen-science.at, https://www.buergerschaffenwissen.de. Accessed on: 6. Febr. 2021
11. Homepage der Scienceslams. https://www.scienceslam.de, http://www.scienceslam.at. Accessed on: 10. Febr. 2021
12. https://www.technischesmuseum.at/besuchen/experimente_fuer_zuhause. Accessed on: 6. Febr. 2021
13. https://ist.ac.at/de/popupscience/. Accessed on: 6. Febr. 2021
14. https://youngscience.at. Accessed on: 6. Febr. 2021
15. https://science-lab.org. Accessed on: 6. Febr. 2021

16. Wikipedia (2021) Kinder- und Jugendanwaltschaft. https://de.wikipedia.org/wiki/Kinder-_und_Jugendanwaltschaft. Accessed on: 6. Febr. 2021
17. Broschüre Kindeswohlgefährdung. https://www.frauen-familien-jugend.bka.gv.at/suchergebnis.html?num=20&q=kindeswohl. Accessed on: 4. Febr. 2021
18. https://www.gewaltinfo.at/recht/mitteilungspflicht/, https://www.dgkim.de/leitlinien/awmf-s3-kinderschutzleitlinie. Accessed on: 4. Febr. 2021
19. Meldeformular für Gefährdungen des Kindeswohls in Österreich. https://www.gewaltinfo.at/uploads/pdf/recht/Meldeformular.pdf. Accessed on: 4. Febr. 2021
20. https://kja.at/site/kinder-in-radikalen-religioesen-gruppen-bericht-einer-aussteigerin-aufruf-zum-hinschauen/. Accessed on: 4. Febr. 2021
21. https://rechtsextremismus-und-familie.de. Accessed on: 6. Febr. 2021
22. Broschüre „Funktionalisierte Kinder" von Andreas Hechler. https://rechtsextremismus-und-familie.de/mediapool/funktionalisierte_kinder_online.pdf. S. 66. Accessed on: 12. Jan. 2020
23. Gollan A, Riede S, Schlang S (2018) Glaubensfreiheit versus Kindeswohl. Familienrechtliche Konflikte im Kontext religiöser und weltanschaulicher Gemeinschaften. Drei-W, Köln

9

Business Life and Professional Training

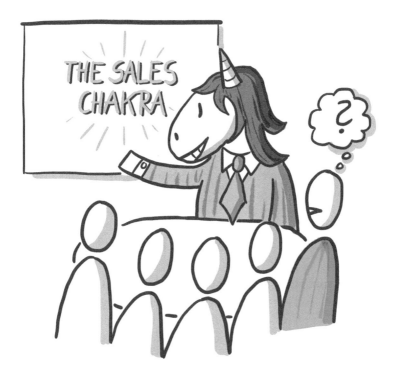

Our boss only hires people who have the astrological sign Libra. They would be the best employees, and since she herself is a Libra, we would get along best that way.

© The Author(s), under exclusive license to Springer-Verlag GmbH, DE, part of Springer Nature 2022
H. G. Hümmler, U. Schiesser, *Fact and Prejudice*, https://doi.org/10.1007/978-3-662-66032-4_9

Our image of business and of people's actions in companies is shaped by the idea of sober profit maximization based on decisions that are as rational as possible. Most of the modeling in economics is based on the idea that economically acting players make at least on average rational decisions. In fact, the reality in many companies is different when looking behind the scenes. Not every entrepreneur is as discreet as the clients of a shaman who advertises on her homepage that employees need not notice when superiors want to *"avail themselves of the help of the spirits"* [1]. A Swiss management consultancy promises to optimize processes in companies by scanning the *"information carriers of the zero point field"* with quantum physical methods [2]. Such a field does not exist in serious physics. Nevertheless, medium-sized entrepreneurs enthusiastically report in the video channel of the consulting company how their business has improved while using the pseudoscientific method [3]. Also, the discussions about graphology in personnel selection, which our fictional Sophie had to conduct in the introductory chapter, are neither unrealistic nor extreme individual cases. The Osnabrück professor of business psychology Uwe Kanning [4] repeatedly points out such questionable methods especially in human resources.

In most cases, we can only slightly influence our working environment and the people we interact with there on a daily basis, but at the same time it is precisely here that we spend most of our time. This field is also dominated by dependencies and power structures like no other. Acting as a critic and admonisher, denouncing unscientific products, rejecting questionable methods and people, can lead to massive personal disadvantages, up to and including the loss of one's job.

9.1   Problem Areas that Can Occur

Colleagues or managers aggressively promote a particular ideology, religion, worldview. You are urged to take a corresponding seminar or coaching. They sell a product on the side, for example in the form of multi-level marketing, which has nothing to do with the field of work. It is particularly difficult to refuse if a manager or a person from the work environment is involved, with whom there is a dependency relationship.

My colleague sends me video links to various conspiracy theories. He is convinced that a collapse of the economy and social order is imminent. He annoys everyone with his warnings that one must arm oneself, buy gold and live as self-sufficiently as possible.

All conversations with him sooner or later revolve around these topics. He is increasingly shunned in the company. I work most closely with him and need a good working relationship with him. I am embarrassed to receive links to dubious right-wing Internet platforms from him via the company e-mail account. I don't want my colleagues to think I approve of that.

***

My advisor at the Federal Employment Agency said that I had an exhausted aura. She asked me if she should do an energy transfer for me. I found the whole thing ridiculous, but I am unemployed, and this woman can cause me considerable problems if she wants to, so I went along with it. But then she recommended seminars to me that she does on the weekends. She said she was actually a "light healer" and saw great potential in me. I don't want to upset this woman, she was otherwise very helpful to me. But how do I get out of this?

Employees are required to attend training courses in the religious or esoteric field.

My boss insisted that I attend a 4-day seminar that is supposed to change my personality in a positive way. It costs a few hundred euros, which I would have to finance myself. However, she has already registered me without asking me and will pay for the flight and accommodation costs. I have read critical reports about the organizer on the Internet and I don't want to do that, but I have only recently been hired through the intervention of my boss and I don't want to put her on the spot.

***

We are a small family business with twelve employees, there are few employers in our region. Recently, the entrepreneurial family has been getting advice from a guru who is increasingly interfering in all matters of the company. The "energy flow" in the company must be optimized, he says. For this purpose, metal plates are installed in every room to provide "positive ionization." In addition, the healer conducts talks and healing rituals with the employees. If I complain, I lose the job, and there are no good alternatives for me.

In recruiting, unscientific methods are used for personnel selection, such as birth charts, handwriting analyses or other unscientific procedures.

In the interview, in addition to my birthday, they asked for my birth time. They would use it to create a "computer chart" that would show my abilities and weaknesses. It was not a horoscope, but a new, allegedly scientific procedure that had been used in this company for a long time with great success.

Contents based on Worldview mix sometimes with factual contents and must be supported.

> *I work as a physician in a group practice. My colleagues increasingly offer treatments and preparations from the alternative medicine sector and want to market this as a focus of the center. It goes down very well with the patients, but I find a lot of it nonsensical and unserious. I don't want to be associated with it, but I don't want to switch the practice because the location is ideal for me.*
>
> ***
>
> *I am a branch manager in a privately owned company. The founder of the company is recently being coached by a person whom he is increasingly in thrall to. He trusts this coach blindly, makes all decisions in the company dependent on his approval, attends expensive seminars with him and also requires employees to attend his seminars at their own expense. The coach acts unprofessionally; the questions he asks are far too personal, manipulative and encroaching. The information is then passed on to the boss. Since I have openly criticized the coach and refuse to attend seminars with him, I have become increasingly isolated and bullied. I was told that my negative attitude was causing an "energetic" effect that would jeopardize the financial success of the company. Positive thinking and an unshakable belief in the boss and his coach would guarantee the success of the company.*

In order to protect employees and customers, the workplace should be kept free of religious, political and ideological propaganda. (Unless it is specifically the field of activity of the company).

> *Of course, an employee can do whatever he/she wants privately, as long as the action is within the legal realm. Employees can also tell colleagues about their private hobbies, views, purchases, etc. during breaks. Employers can intervene if the agreed work performance is not fulfilled or if other employees feel harassed or threatened. In this case, the employer is even obligated to intervene due to his duty of care towards the other employees. What can employers do in this case? They can issue instructions and warnings, hold discussions with employees, inform superiors … But only if a certain potential for harassment has been reached.* (Doris Rauscher-Kalod, Head of the Department of Labor and Social Law, Chamber of Labor for Lower Austria).

Company training must be related to the job, paid for by the employer and can be completed during working hours. If employees carry out a secondary commercial activity, it must be clarified whether this is permitted under the employment contract. Sometimes non-competition clauses prohibit additional earnings for one's own business, or they must at least be approved by the employer. In all cases, however, the rule applies again that working hours and work equipment may not be used for additional income.

A particular problem that can arise in discussions with representatives of unscientific belief systems, especially in companies, is what coach Peter Modler calls *"vertical communication"* [5]. In business, more than in other areas of our lives, professional discussions often involve issues of status, power, and hierarchy in addition to the actual content. Whereas in horizontal communication, which is largely independent of hierarchy, factual arguments are in the foreground, vertical communication is primarily concerned with establishing and securing rankings. Modler attributes Donald Trump's temporary great success in politics to the fact that he succeeded in asserting his form of vertical communication in political discourse, which was unusual and difficult for his opponents to attack. Thus, when the personnel manager insists on a graphological assessment of applicants, it is not only a matter of his enthusiasm for this pseudo-scientific instrument, but always also of preserving his position as an expert decision-maker in personnel selection.

This does not mean that content and factual arguments play no role in vertical communication. However, they are usually in the foreground as long as there is no conflict. In the event of conflict, vertical communication quickly shifts to concise, highly simplified or generalized statements that are difficult to counter at the content level. In addition, positioning in space plays a special role in vertical communication, which can reflect differences in rank, distance, ignoring, but also deliberately unpleasant closeness.

In the following fictitious example of vertical communication, the genders of the actors are not chosen at random, because traditional images of "masculinity" play just as much a role in vertical communication as do actual or informal hierarchies. So let us return once again to her workplace with Sophie from the introduction:

> Sophie and her colleague Mr. Groß are sitting, their laptops in front of them on the table, in a meeting with other employees of the company and discussing their different interpretations of the latest market research data. Both initially justify their position from the data. When Mr. Groß is unable to assert himself in terms of content, he repeats his last argument and concludes with the terse, pointed statement: "That's the way it is."

If Sophie now continues to stay on the level of factual arguments, Mr. Groß will not respond. What is worse, however, is that even colleagues who are sympathetic to her will no longer concern themselves with her factual arguments, but rather with the question of how she reacts to this confrontation.

If, however, she changes to the same level, for example with a spirited *"That's what you say!"* and endures the tense pause that is likely to result, then she has a chance that the discussion will subsequently return to factual arguments. However, it could also happen that Mr. Groß escalates the situation further by getting up and standing behind Sophie, ostensibly to discuss data on her screen. In doing so, he demonstratively violates the rules of a polite distance on the one hand, and on the other hand, he literally places himself above her. A discussion about factual arguments is thus no longer possible. As a counter-strategy, Sophie could either also stand up and bend over her computer together with Mr. Groß, or she could demonstratively pull out a chair for him. In both cases, the literal eye level would be restored before talking about content again.

Non-verbal forms of vertical communication express themselves not only in momentary behaviors, but also, for example, in things like office furnishings or clothing. For example, soccer coaches who wear similar training clothes to their players at games or press conferences are regularly seen by the public as more affable but less capable of leadership than those who show up to such appointments in suits.

Food for Thought

Have you ever felt the urge to act as a missionary for your personal convictions in your professional environment, even if this was not appropriate in terms of content? Are there people who are in a relationship of dependence to you and who cannot easily tell you that they want to be left alone? Have you yourself ever had the "pleasure" of unwanted religious, spiritual, ideological or political propaganda in business life? How do you then react to this harassment as an employee, manager or customer?

The professional problem cases in relation to dubious offers and esotericism are often small and family businesses. If the couple who run the carpentry shop in hicksville are enamored of a guru, it is far more difficult for employees to distance themselves than in a large corporation where, for example, help and advice can be sought from the works council.

9.2 Being Affected as a Colleague

Seek a clarifying discussion, which should be conducted in a factual and constructive manner. In the case of unscientific products and processes, refer to articles in scientific journals and reputable online sources. Place value on good sources of information and also demand reputable sources for claims from the counterpart. Attempt a factual discourse about the claimed causes and effects first. It may be useful to clarify in advance whether other colleagues share your opinion. You will achieve more if you act as a group and not just as the lone voice in the wilderness. Especially when superiors advocate unscientific products or processes, it strengthens your position enormously if you are supported in your arguments by colleagues. Together you can achieve more; an individual can be defamed more quickly as a troublemaker and isolated.

An important argument for companies is always the public image. One wants to be seen as a serious, reliable company that does not become the laughing stock of competitors or even receive negative press coverage.

An example is the company Sonnentor, which has made a name for itself in the organic food sector with the production of spices and teas. Due to customer requests, in 2007 they began to add a horizontal line to the barcode on their products. In esoteric circles, there is an idea among some that the barcode transmits negative vibrations from the environment to the product and then, amplified by the scanner at the checkout, has a harmful effect on health [6]. In 2013, this practice was pointed out in a mailing list of the Viennese skeptics, the Society for Critical Thinking (GkD), whereupon a number of outraged customers communicated their anger to the Sonnentor company. Critical blog posts and newspaper articles followed [7].

Florian Aigner summed up why assertions of this kind are not only nonsense, but also harmful [8]:

> One must never forget with such theories: There are people who actually believe in them. There are people who suffer from this belief, who dare not buy barcode-printed products anymore, who actually get physical pain due to a strong nocebo effect. Those who promote such abstruse, scientifically completely untenable theories by even making them seem possible are helping to increase this suffering.

Sonnentor reacted quickly to this criticism and stopped "suppressing" the barcode. The company's press spokeswoman at the time, Manuela Seebacher, commented in an interview on why the horizontal bar was originally printed [9]:

> To be honest, not much thought was put into it. There was simply no extra effort. It also wasn't actively communicated and brought to the public. There are a few companies that do that; we weren't the only ones. But it wasn't that big of an issue; we just didn't deal with it in such detail. We just wanted to allay some people's fears. [...] Now there was a lot of feedback from customers who didn't want that. Many felt that unfounded fears were being stoked and a misconception was being pro-

moted. The topic has polarized, so we looked into it more intensively, and we concluded that barcode suppression does not fit Sonnentor. I think it's important to stick to your line and stand by it.

This example shows how unreflectively companies sometimes engage in promotions. A vague customer interest and a few employees who share this ideology are often enough for a company to support nonsensical measures. Disgruntled customers, the threat of loss of face in the industry and negative reporting can quickly lead to a change of mind. Use your influence as a consumer.

When I'm in a hotel that boasts of using Grander water[1] I always complain to the front desk about it. They should realize that they are losing my respect and sympathy. In a restaurant that advertises on its menu that all water is energized with the Grander system, I have told them that I am not allowed to drink Grander water for religious reasons. It would be esoteric and therefore forbidden for me as a Christian. It is not true for me, but I want to point out that they do not automatically make all customers happy with such an offer.[2]

Back to the discussion with colleagues and superiors: It may be that your counterpart does not want to engage in a factual discussion or that it is about an ideology and worldview that is not amenable to arguments, for example, if a colleague is an anti-vaxxer, a member of a cult-like community or of the freemen movement and is proselytizing in the company and with customers. In this case, don't waste too much time discussing the value, truth or content of a worldview/religion, but stick to the impact on the work environment. Make it clear that you feel harassed by the proselytizing attempts and that you fear a negative impact on the company.

If the counterpart uses the above-mentioned means of vertical communication, it is first of all helpful to recognize when they occur and to understand that you can hardly counter them by remaining only on the content level yourself. At worst, an accumulation of factual arguments is then reinterpreted as justification or excuse. When dealing with dominant men, coach Peter Modler recommends that women respond to concise, pointed statements with their own concise, pointed statements, and to positioning in the room with positioning in the room – at least until one has reached an equality of means and can return to the factual level [5]. In the example above, Sophie

---

[1] Water supposedly "energized" by a para-scientific process.
[2] Some free churches outlaw any consumption of and contact with esoteric products, as they are frowned upon as "witchcraft" and "the work of Satan".

could have done this in dealing with her dominant colleague Mr. Groß. This does not only work if one is officially equal or in the hierarchically better position. With superiors, it can be quite helpful to explicitly acknowledge the hierarchical differences they mark: *"You are the head of department"* acknowledges authority, but also insinuates who may be responsible for an ordered seminar for the entire team with a questionable motivational trainer. Whether this would have helped Sophie in dealing with the graphology-believing personnel manager from the introduction, however, cannot be clearly predicted, of course. Even models such as vertical communication only ever depict individual aspects of the complex processes in a discussion.

If available, turn to anonymous complaint bodies, the works council, the trade union. Sometimes, however, it is necessary to first raise awareness of the problem, because managers or members of the works council may themselves be proponents of a problematic offer. Such problem cases are also too rarely reported to employee representatives, chambers and trade unions. The attitude that *"there's nothing we can do about it anyway"* prevents awareness of this problem area from developing and prevents company agreements and legal regulations from being adapted in the longer term.

Keep an eye on how ideology can affect clients and job projects. The home health aide who offers Archangel Gabriel drops for high blood pressure to her clients can do significant damage to both her charges and the company's reputation. The sales representative who also warns about the dangers of 5G and tells about QAnon at every customer meeting is damaging his own reputation and that of his company. This employee may be acting in well-meaning good faith and without realizing how detrimental his or her involvement can be.

9.3 Responsibility as Company Management

If you have management responsibility in the company, then it makes sense to determine a general handling of ideological offers. If an employee distributes advertising material in the company, it makes sense not only to argue why exactly this guru, this community, this political movement may not be distributed via professional networks, but to formulate a general policy of the company on all comparable offers. For example, a supermarket or a pharmacy should establish a basic line on which folders may be displayed in the store and which advertising posters may be hung. That objectifies the argumentation, why e.g. coworker A may put out an invitation for autogenic training, but coworker B not the one for his spiritual healer circle.

For educational institutions, universities, seminar houses and the like, this demarcation is particularly important, since the place where an event takes place or the provider of a lecture or seminar can already convey respectability. Examples are: The guru yoga group that offers meditation courses for UN employees and henceforth calls itself a cooperation partner of the UN; the pseudo-scientific bioresonance offer that rents university premises for a conference and thus gives itself an apparently scientific veneer; the recognized educational institute of the Chamber of Commerce that also offers courses on aura reading.

The Austrian Adult Education Centers (Volkshochschulen) have, to give a positive example, the basic guideline not to include unscientific content in their course program – a not uncontroversial position, since there is great demand for courses on esotericism and alternative medicine, and they are a "customer magnet". This demarcation is clearly formulated [10]:

> *The adult education center is thus not a place for the dissemination of doctrines of salvation and anti-democratic world views. It does not provide a platform for propaganda, agitation, product advertising or for the recruitment of "clientele" by political, religious or other ideological groups. Thus, there are limits to openness and diversity – in the sense of arbitrariness.* (Recommendation for the design of educational work at adult education centers).

In order to establish quality criteria in the mushrooming offer of adult education, standards were formulated and procedures for the evaluation of providers were developed. Ö-Zert represents a quality seal of this kind. In the guidelines for applicants, the distinction between adult education and esotericism is formulated as follows [11]:

> *No theory disputes that education has to do with forming a critical consciousness on the basis of and through the rational examination of knowledge that is currently regarded as secure, and with acquiring personally, professionally and socially relevant and secure knowledge for action. When talking about education, it is ultimately always about thinking and acting on one's own responsibility towards oneself, nature and society. Education is therefore not compatible with the uncritical transmission of ideologies, allegedly unquestionable secret knowledge or belief systems.*
>
> *Educational events can only fulfill their immanent promise if they focus on imparting scientifically recognized knowledge and promoting the ability to enable participants to engage in rational and critical debate and to act on this knowledge.*

Fundamental specifications, with elaborated criteria, should also be in place to ensure the quality of professional training offers, coaching, etc. Internal company standards protect employees from arbitrariness and appropriation. That also helps budget responsibles to decide which further training offers should be supported. These criteria can also be applied when employees ask for (additional) funding for continuing education programs.

Takeaway

Business life, which is misunderstood as rational, is also susceptible to promises of success from dubious providers and unscientific products. In one's own company, acting as a critic and admonisher against this is particularly delicate due to the dependency and power structures in this field. Support from like-minded people, a look at the external impact on customers and the company's reputation, as well as basic regulations for dealing with religious/spiritual/ideological offerings can be helpful. Educational institutions have a special responsibility not to give controversial methods the appearance of respectability.

References

1. Ferreiro P (2012) Schamanische Unternehmensberatung. http://www.tunkash-ila.eu/index.php?option=com_content&view=article&id=17&Itemid=7. Accessed on: 11. Dez. 2020
2. Fretz B (2017) Scannen + Informieren. https://www.fretz-partner.ch/unternehmensberatung-zuerich-unternehmensberatung-mit-quantenphysik-3/scannen-informieren. Accessed on: 19. Dez. 2020
3. Fretz B (2020) Unternehmensphysiker wie geht das? https://www.youtube.com/channel/UCA8muf-C3ZQnDJnk9FjsGHg/videos. Accessed on: 19. Dez. 2020
4. Kanning UP (2015) Personalauswahl zwischen Anspruch und Wirklichkeit. Springer, Heidelberg
5. Modler P (2019) Mit Ignoranten sprechen. Campus, Frankfurt a.M
6. https://www.psiram.com/de/index.php/Strichcode-Verschwörung. Accessed on: 1. Mai 2021
7. https://www.derstandard.at/story/1369363223244/gefaehrlicher-barcode, https://www.faz.net/aktuell/gesellschaft/gesundheit/barcode-bedenken-das-kreuz-mit-den-strichen-12133019.html. Accessed on: 1. Mai 2021
8. https://scienceblogs.de/naklar/2013/06/02/faule-kompromisse/. Accessed on: 1. Mai 2021
9. https://www.biorama.eu/barcode-entstorung-ein-strich-durch-die-striche/. Accessed on: 1. Mai 2021
10. https://www.vhs.or.at/538/. Accessed on: 1. Mai 2021
11. https://oe-cert.at/media/leitfaden.pdf. Accessed on: 1. Mai 2021

10

Health Care and Social System

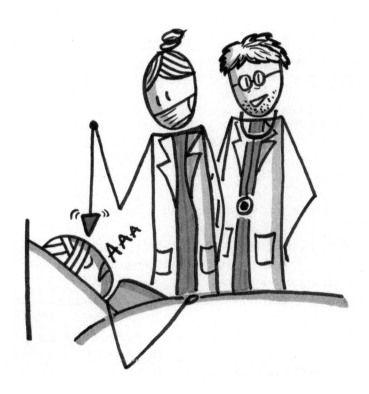

H. G. Hümmler, U. Schiesser, *Fact and Prejudice*,
https://doi.org/10.1007/978-3-662-66032-4_10

10.1   The Medical Field

My mother (63 years old) has severe hip pain. She was scheduled for surgery to have a hip joint replaced. Several people in our circle of acquaintances have already had this surgery and are thrilled with how well they feel since then. My mother knows this, but still canceled the surgery a week before. Her condition is deteriorating, she can hardly walk longer distances. She relies on a Brazilian spiritual healer to care for her remotely. Three times a day she takes herbal pills prescribed by this spiritual healer. The content of these pills is unknown, on the package it says only "Archangel Michael."

***

My best friend is overweight and has a heart condition for which he must take medication. He is in thrall to a woman who calls herself a witch and has persuaded him that his illness is only psychological because he died in a previous life as a Roman soldier from a spear thrust to the heart. She sets the dosage of his medication daily, with the help of a pendulum.

***

Professionally, I have also repeatedly had to deal with terminally ill people and their relatives. Often enough, people were confronted with hopeless diagnoses overnight. Their reactions and those of their relatives were very different. Some accepted their fate. Others began to fight for their recovery. Often enough I was able to witness, which is all too understandable, how people in this situation grasped at every straw that offered itself for salvation. And the straws were blown by the wind of alternative, complementary and holistic miracle healing. Nobody dies in these sympathetic ordinations. But the terminally ill are treated only until they are out of treatment. Then they are handed back to the family doctor. This is precisely the time when life really comes to an end. The family doctor is then allowed to care for his patients until death. (Edmund Berndt, pharmacist and author)

Today, health care professionals are faced with a number of challenges: high demands on professional education and training, framework conditions that make personal conversations, relationship work and the intensive care of individual patients very difficult, and patients who increasingly act as demanding consumers and also use various more or less reputable sources of information. Despite constantly improving treatment methods and clear successes, for example in cancer treatment, there is skepticism towards "orthodox/western/mainstrem medicine" (the problematic term "Schulmedizin") [1] to the point of strict rejection. In the environment of esotericism those voices became louder and louder in the last decade, which advise against medical treatments, reject medicines and accuse the whole health sector of unfair motives and unfair practices. In extreme cases, conspiracy myths are spread: *"Doctors and pharmaceutical companies are part of the world conspiracy that really wants to make us sick and control us."*

In friendlier terms, it is formulated, for example, like this: *"Every illness is an expression of a psychological conflict or an energy imbalance. Medical treatments only relieve the symptoms, but do not solve the basic problem. Only method XY can do that. Therefore, only method XY must be applied."*

Where many esoteric healing procedures used to parallel medical treatment, there are now increasing claims of a superiority of these concepts and discouragement of necessary evidence-based treatments. *"When you go to a hospital (in German "Krankenhaus" literally translated means "house of the sick"), the very word tells you that you must be sick in that place. You're creating a resonance in the universe that creates illness in the first place. That's why diagnoses are harmful. They make you sick because they tell you that you are sick."* By the way, using this logic, one client cancelled her health insurance (in German "sick insurance") because it would signal to the universe that she was afraid for her health. The universe – seemingly endowed with a simple mind – would then promptly deliver exactly what one fears: Illness. Canceling the insurance would instead signal to the universe how confident the person was in remaining invulnerable and healthy. Impressed by this act of self-confidence, the universe would then deliver to one exactly what was ordered.

Why do people, even in the case of life-threatening diseases, turn away from functioning medical treatments and seek their salvation with sometimes dubious providers? Because elementary human needs are given too little attention in modern everyday medical life: the longing for attention, compassion, touch; the desire to confide in a reliable person who gives comfort and hope. For some, there is a childlike longing to hand over responsibility for one's own suffering to someone else, only to be healed effortlessly, and without any change in lifestyle [2]. Others are particularly concerned in stressful situations to retain as much control as possible; they need a lot of information and want to be involved in all decisions. All of this demands a lot of time, empathy, and skills in conversation from medical professionals. These are precisely the needs that are the focus of the alternative and esoteric provider sector. The better emotional care trumps the expert medical treatment; to the patients this is also worth a lot of money. Edzard Ernst, who dedicates himself in his scientific activity to the research of alternative and natural medicine, notes: *"Overall, the impression is that the current popularity of alternative medicine is in some ways also a sharp critique of the shortcomings of today's conventional health care."* [3]

People want someone who will take the time. Scientific medicine has been econo-mized; psychotherapy and pediatricians are paid the least. Conversation has been pushed further and further into the background over the last 25 years. (Thomas F, pediatrician)

For the German profession "Heilpraktiker" (naturopath) there is no state pre-scribed uniform qualification. There are different extensive trainings, which are not subject to any state regulation and can be completed voluntarily. A prerequisite for admission as a non-medical practitioner is the granting of a license, which, in addition to formal criteria, provides for a "clearance test", a written and oral test of knowledge and skills, which may be repeated as often as desired if the test is not passed. The test is not a specific level of training, but whether the person could be a danger to the health of others. Heilpraktiker are allowed to diagnose and treat on their own responsibility; only the use of prescription drugs, obstetrics and treatment of infectious diseases are prohib-ited. In Austria, there is no comparable professional profile; a healing treat-ment may only be performed by doctors.

Alternative therapists and providers in the esoteric sector can be much more uninhibited in promising healing, which will often not happen in seri-ous medical care. The danger is that they fall victim to the Dunning-Kruger effect:[1] They overestimate their competence, their own experience, and their ability to cure illness. Since this lack of self-criticism endows them with great self-confidence, they appear very convincing to those seeking help, and they are trusted to deliver what they promise [4]. An improvement in health is then also attributed to their actions rather than to the natural healing process and other treatments taking place at the same time.

However, dissatisfaction with working conditions or treatment methods also exists within the medical professions themselves. Then doctors, nurses, midwives etc. turn to alternative concepts. These can serve as a helpful supple-ment, as an attempt to better meet the needs of the sick, but can also go along with a skeptical attitude towards academic medicine among this group of people.

In the healthcare field, conflicts arise in two main ways: Either you are a scientifically oriented person working in this field and are confronted with patients who hold a different worldview, or you are a patient yourself and are recommended treatments that are not evidence-based.

---

[1] Dunning-Kruger effect: incompetent people overestimate their knowledge precisely because they do not have enough information to critically assess themselves and perceive their limitations.

Help, My Doctor Is a Shaman!

I had been having colds on and off for months and was feeling listless, so I went to the new family doctor in the building next door. She seemed competent to me, she listened to me, took her time and seemed to have a good grasp of my problem. And then suddenly came the sentence I dread the most: "We can well do something homeopathic there." Now there are two possibilities: Either she thinks my problem is psychosomatic and just needs a placebo, in which case I don't feel taken seriously by her. Or she really believes that little balls of sugar will make me well, in which case I can't take her seriously.

***

I have often found it not so easy to tell a doctor (preferably right from the start) that I don't think much of alternative methods. Nor do I feel like listening to a doctor's "good experiences" with non-evidence based stuff. Now I have been trying the following method for some time: During the anamnesis, at some point the question inevitably comes up, "Do you have any allergies or intolerances?" To which I answer, "Homeopathy, Bach flowers and Grander water."

The best answer so far: "Are you also allergic to holy water?" (Gabriele Imrich-Schwarz)
***

I always inform myself well about the diagnosis and possible procedures. If a doctor suggests a treatment that does not seem serious to me, I ask for a detailed explanation of the mechanism of action. That's when you can quickly tell how well he or she knows and whether they are comprehensible and scientific concepts. Certain terms are warnings: Energy flow, fields, meridians, detoxification. (Michael Mikas)

The mailing lists of the GWUP (German sceptics society) are regularly engaged with the question if it is not possible to create a list of health professionals who do not use esoteric methods, do not recommend homeopathy, are evidence-based in their treatment and keep up to date with new findings in research and development. Addresses of these doctors, physiotherapists, midwives, etc. are highly sought after. Why is it not self-evident that a doctor uses evidence-based methods?

Here is a joke:

A physics student, a mathematics student and a medical student are each presented with a phone book by their professors. The physics student: *"I cannot infer the experiment from these measurement results, and thus the result is too inaccurate and worthless!"* The mathematics student: *"These numbers cannot be summarized as a mathematical series, thus they are definitions by definition. And without context, these definitions are worthless."* The medical student just looks wearily at the professor and asks: *"By when am I supposed to memorize these?"* [5]

This joke parodies the experience that medical school does not place as much emphasis on teaching critical thinking and critical questioning of one's own field. The basics of statistics, design of scientific studies, and the field of philosophy of science also have little value in the curriculum. Later, in practical training, the hierarchical structures in hospitals mean that dubious methods of treatment are adopted without being questioned.

The entire system of medical training, especially for junior physicians, is hierarchical. Ultimately, this leads to the fact that as a junior you do what your superior says, and criticism is not welcome, and one thinks to oneself, they have dealt with this, they know what they are doing, otherwise they would not be a senior physician or a chief physician. With some things, it was not at all obvious how unscientific it all was. I took over a lot. (Florian Albrecht, physician)

***

I have never seen any treatment success with homeopathy. Not with me and not with my patients. I thought to myself, I am the mistake, the others are doing a great job. There were only three options at meetings of homeopaths: It's the right medicine because it gets better; it's the right medicine because it gets worse at first, or it's the wrong medicine. (Thomas F., pediatrician)

Even experienced physicians easily fall into the trap of relying too much on their own clinical experience. This overlooks the fact that this experience can be distorted by biases: The natural course of the disease, the placebo effect, the effect of the doctor-patient relationship, confirmation bias, and other effective factors influence the success of a treatment [3]. The validity of individual cases is easily overestimated, especially because there are often pre-assumptions about treatment methods that also influence the perception of effects. Ideally, evidence-based medicine should complement and objectify clinical experience with reliable evidence. For this, it is necessary to approach one's own perception with a critical caution. However, many patients place less weight on treatment than on the time, attention, and emotional support they receive from the clinician [3].

Unfortunately, medical education, at least for physicians, is still grossly deficient: The personal conversation, the psychological factors of the treatment and the relationship as well as placebo and nocebo effects are hardly taught in the studies. In everyday clinical practice, there is usually a lack of time and appreciation for this aspect of care. Often, those health professionals who are interested in alternative or esoteric treatments are also particularly dedicated. They invest time and money in additional training and seek ways to better care for their patients. Many feel hindered by the health care system in this endeavor. Frustrated, some develop a clear rejection of standard medical practice and position themselves as an alternative or in opposition to it. Others add various non-evidence-based procedures as tools of treatment to conventional ones. It is very difficult for patients to distinguish one from the other.

The well-known physician and author Eckart von Hirschhausen suggests patients to ask the following five questions before any treatment [2]:

1. What is the benefit?
2. What are the risks?
3. Where is the evidence?
4. What happens if we wait and watch?
5. Would you do what you recommend yourself?

For information on the effectiveness of a healing procedure, there are a number of **reputable medical online sites** available (in German):

- gesund.bund.de
- gutepillen-schlechtepillen.de
- www.gesundheitsinformation.de
- www.bzga.de
- www.weisse-liste.de
- www.gesundheit.gv.at
- wissenwaswirkt.org
- www.patienten-information.de
- www.stiftung-gesundheitswissen.de
- www.medizin-transparent.at
- www.igel-monitor.de
- www.krebsinformationsdienst.de
- www.infonetz-krebs.de
- www.psychenet.de/de/
- de.wikipedia.org/wiki/Psiram
- selpers.com
- www.krankheitserfahrungen.de

- English: www.hon.ch/en/
- **App:** medbusters.at

How can you judge the **quality of an online site**? "Medizin-Transparent" (Cochrane Austria) recommends the following criteria for health sites on the Internet [6]:

1. No advertising
2. Author information instead of anonymity
3. Date of last update
4. Scientific references
5. Neutral, non-judgmental language
6. Addressing disadvantages
7. Mentioning other treatments
8. Is the treatment physically perceptible?
9. Concrete numbers and comparisons
10. How well backed up is the research?

In the appendix of the book you will find further sources of serious medical information. Also recommended are the books by Edzard Ernst, who has studied the effectiveness of alternative healing methods for many years. "Alternative Medicine: A Critical Assessment of 150 Modalities" summarizes the results of this research and describes the effectiveness of 150 alternative treatment concepts.

Takeaway

When personal health is at stake, people are especially susceptible to promises of quick, easy and comprehensive cures. This is also where the greatest damage is done when unprofessional providers overestimate themselves. The need for wholeness, for being seen and cared for as a person in all aspects, for time and attention, is particularly great for the sick. This is seldom possible in the medical business; therefore, health professionals also like to switch to alternative and not always reputable forms of treatment. As a patient, remain critical of healing methods that promise a lot, advertise primarily with case histories, and are not evidence-based.

Help, My Patient Is Superstitious!

I have often asked people who have suffered for decades from chronic, non-curable conditions such as psoriasis, ankylosing spondylitis, etc. about their treatment careers. The common tenor of the answers was that it had taken about 5 to 10 years until they had finally understood literally from bad experience that there is nothing to the many wonderful healing promises and the "simple" explanations for the causes of disease of the alternative, complementary and holistic miracle healers. Over time, they said, they had come to realize that they were better off with their ailment in conventional medicine. Of course, they had also made both good and bad experiences here, but they would now no longer run after any healing promise, no matter how great. (Edmund Berndt, pharmacist and author)

In Lower Austria, a 13-year-old girl died of chronic pancreatitis in September 2019 after years of suffering. The parents, who were members of a fundamental Christian free church, had only prayed until the end, trusting that God would heal the child. Medical treatment was not sought. The diagnosis had been made during a hospitalization two years earlier, with a strong warning that ongoing medical care was imperative. The family seemed to have had a very negative experience of their time in the hospital; their stay there was prematurely terminated, and further treatment was not sought. The parents seemed convinced to the end that they were doing the right thing for their child [7].

This very drastic example shows how far-reaching the consequences can be when people assume alternative cause-and-effect principles. Something similar is known from Jehovah's Witnesses, who persistently refuse blood transfusions even if there is a danger to life – in this case not because the effect of the treatment is doubted, but because with the intake of foreign blood not only an irrevocable spiritual damage is feared, but also disobedience to God's laws would be shown. It is accepted to die prematurely in this earthly life in order not to lose the chance of an eternal life in paradise. The basis of this attitude of faith are Bible passages such as the following: *"abstain from things polluted by idols, from sexual immorality, from what is strangled, and from blood."* (Acts 15:19–20) [8].

Identifying fundamental beliefs in patients is an important first step in being able to discuss them at all. Religion and worldview are too rarely addressed in healthcare. This area is usually only considered in terms of respecting religious rules; positive and negative impact factors of the respective faith are rarely questioned. Particular attention should be paid to this influence on underage patients. Here there is also a social responsibility to put the welfare of the child before the religious freedom of the parents [9].

Arthur Kleinman, professor of medical anthropology and cross-cultural psychiatry at Harvard University, has dealt with cultural differences in concepts of illness. He argues that an illness always includes the dimension of a personal experience and explanation of illness, and that we develop a personal narrative[2] of our condition that is effective in how we feel and in the treatment we provide. To make this personal illness narrative visible and understandable, he formulated the following eight questions:

1. What do you call your problem?
2. What do you think caused your problem?

---

[2] A story that we develop to make sense of the world.

3. Why do you think it started when it did?
4. What do you think your sickness does to you? How does it work?
5. How severe is it? Will it have a short or long course?
6. What do you fear most about your disorder?
7. What are the chief problems your sickness has caused for you?
8. What have you done so far to treat your illness? What treatments do you think you should receive? What are the most important results you hope to receive from the treatment?

These questions are useful not only if the patient is a Chinese rice farmer and one can possibly assume different cultural worldviews, but especially if there is a spiritual/esoteric worldview. For example, if someone believes that their illness was caused by sin and will only get better through repentance, prayer, and the divine blessing, this has far-reaching implications. In this case, social stigma in the patient's environment can lead to late diagnosis, hiding the illness out of shame, and half-hearted treatment or no treatment at all.

Tips for talking to patients

- Do not ridicule or aggressively attack alternative disease concepts – this is more likely to achieve the opposite. Ask exactly which methods patients are using and from which practitioners; ask about the practitioners' training. If you are not familiar with a method or if it does not appear to be serious, let them know. The representatives of a method often present it as recognized, scientifically proven and widely used, even if it is in no way so. Your professional assessment can be an important guide, as long as you do not provoke a defensive attitude in your counterpart.
- If you notice that your counterpart reacts skeptically or pejoratively, address this directly and ask why.
- You yourself as a person are an effective factor in the treatment. The time, attention and empathy that you devote to patients can support healing just as much as the confidence that you radiate, the calm and security that you convey.
- Especially when a disease is first diagnosed and at crucial points in treatment, patients are in an exceptional situation. Even casually said sentences can take on a special weight and act as a suggestion [10]. The anesthesiologist Christel Bejenke warns doctors not to say sentences like *"You will now be put to sleep"* before an operation; most people have negative associations with this. Bejenke [11] recommends the following

wording: *"An anesthesiologist will give you your anesthesia; anesthesia has to do with relaxation, well-being, and safety. And the anesthesiologist will stay with you and ensure your safety while you are completely relaxed."* Hearing the phrase "It's all over" after surgery can create anxiety, whereas hearing the phrase "Your surgery is done, everything is fine with you" is reassuring and supportive [12]. Your words create a placebo or nocebo effect and are a very effective part of your treatment; precise and careful phrasing is essential. For example, when you refer to a relapse as a lap of honor, you create other associations and support self-efficacy and hope. This does not mean trivializing problems and lying to patients; the statements must be realistic prognoses. However, this still gives leeway in the form of communication.

- A good concluding question of the anamnesis can be: *"Is there anything else I should know so I can take good care of you?"*
- Things said are better understood, remembered and believed if you use visual aids to support the message. Use visuals, anatomical models, graphics, photos, and pictorial metaphors.
- Ask if other procedures are used and/or various products consumed in parallel with your treatment. *"Please tell me if you are taking other remedies and using other procedures, even if you suspect I don't think anything of it. Maybe you are right about that, maybe I surprise you, but I want to prevent unwanted interactions in any case. This can also happen with natural remedies. For example, St. John's wort oil has a proven effect on depression, but it affects the efficacy of contraceptives and diabetes medications, among other things."* Expect patients to not mention concurrent interventions on their own. In the case of natural remedies, people often naively assume that what is "natural" is fundamentally harmless; in the case of esoteric procedures, they want to avoid incomprehension and ridicule.
- Address possible motives: *"I can understand that you would like to have the gentlest, most natural treatment possible. Perhaps we can combine the two."*
- A sentence like. *"That's bullshit, don't do that!"* will automatically elicit resistance. If it's low impact but harmless: *"I expect little help, but no harm from it either. Just please be careful that no one is profiteering from your condition. It's enough to have your body struggle; it doesn't have to hit your wallet, too."* For procedures that are hazardous to your health: *"I'm worried about you. This could be really dangerous, and you have enough stress as it is."*

- Let patients participate in decisions: When they make a choice from treatment alternatives, after appropriate education, compliance increases and so does the likelihood that they will follow through with treatment consistently. Illness creates a painful feeling of helplessness. Every small decision that can be made is reassuring and restores a sense of control.
- Bring in your own experience: If you yourself have a particular health problem and are taking a particular medication, or someone in your family is, your recommendations are especially credible. *"I faced this decision just like you did, and I chose XY."* Also helpful is the reference: *"If I were in your shoes, I would do XY"* or. *"If it were my child, I would, …"*
- Explain the mode of action of a medication. Explain why a patient should take this particular medication. This may be obvious to you, but probably not to your patient.
- Set common goals. In rehabilitation, for example, better results are achieved if the goals are concrete and relevant to the patient, such as being able to reach the top shelf of the kitchen.
- Is the patient still receptive? Especially during the initial diagnosis, many people are in an exceptional situation, excited and overwhelmed. Their information is only partially absorbed. *"Can you still follow me? I know it's a lot at first, and you can take your time digesting it all first, and if you still have questions, call me and we'll discuss it later."*
- The vast amount of information on health topics available to everyone on the Internet has not necessarily resulted in better informed people. Information is still better absorbed when it is conveyed by a trusted person in a direct conversation.

The Salzburg cardiologist and director of a rehabilitation center, Hans Altenberger, sees the time factor as the linchpin for good patient care:

> During rounds, I only have 5 to 10 minutes for each patient. If I notice that I haven't reached someone, I offer to take time in the afternoon to talk to them. If I notice the person disagrees, I address that as well, "You're not convinced now?" It doesn't bother me if patients have a different opinion; I encourage them to voice it. I explain to patients where I get my information from. If I notice that the factual level is no longer sufficient, then I ask the question of trust: "I have been dealing with this disease for years. I could also make it easier for myself and not spend so much time on this conversation, but it is important to me to take good care of you. You have to decide if you trust me.

***

I have gotten into the habit of using everyday language and speaking as simply as possible. Some find that too banal, then I can raise the tempo and challenge people. (Thomas F., pediatrician)

***

I print out information material for patients that they can understand. In the case of Ayurvedic or Chinese medicine, I advise that they ask the person who prescribes them where they get them from and how safe the standard of these preparations is. If they are produced in Europe, they at least meet certain quality standards; if they come from China or India, they often contain dangerous levels of heavy metals. I have at least fulfilled my duty to inform; I will often not be able to achieve more. Saying, "That's no use, leave it, it's not scientifically proven," is rarely successful. (Florian Albrecht, physician)

***

It is important not to confuse empathy for the patient with telling them what they want to hear. Empathy simply means, I try to understand the patient, his background and his wishes first and foremost. Explanations at eye level can only succeed if you understand your counterpart and know what his or her intentions are. Then you can propose medically sensible solutions that fit the patient's needs. For true patient autonomy, it is important that he or she makes decisions on an informed basis. If a patient then says that he still wants to take the globules, then he should do so in God's name. But if someone comes up with the idea of treating a cancer or a serious illness with homeopathics, then of course a dangerous boundary has been crossed, and then it is also important that as a doctor one points out quite clearly the limits of this sham therapy. (Christian Lübbers, ENT physician)

***

When patients ask for homeopathic products, I say, "Do you want something homeopathic or something that helps?" I then explain that homeopathy is not herbal medicine, that is usually enough. People's need is to use a herbal remedy instead of a pharmaceutical one, and that's where I can support them. (Florian Albrecht, physician)

***

As a doctor, you want to convey factual information, but people are not interested in that at all. Ultimately, it all works on an emotional basis, but you don't learn that in training, you acquire it over time through trial and error. You have to recognize: What is the need of the other person? (Thomas F., pediatrician)

Takeaway

Patients' perceptions of disease affect their willingness to undergo treatment. Despite the abundance of information on the Internet, the personal conversation remains the most important instrument for orientation. Comprehensible language, explanation of contexts and the support of visual material promote trust. As the person treating the patient, you are an effective factor in healing through verbal and nonverbal communication. Involve patients in decisions as often as possible and set common goals. This promotes willingness to cooperate and restores a sense of control.

10.2 Psychology, Psychotherapy, Counseling, Coaching

After 20 years of marriage, my husband and I lost sight of each other a bit. We had few arguments, but hardly spent any time together. Sex was also rather infrequent and more of a chore. We decided to change that in couples therapy. The therapist had all this described to her, then she said she had to "connect with the field," closed her eyes, and made a strange grimace. After a few minutes she looked at us and said, "No wonder you have these problems. You were siblings in the previous life, and of course that is still having an effect. There needs to be a karmic cleansing." We were stunned.

The Gretchen Question[3] "Now tell me, how do you feel about religion?" is often a taboo subject in therapy and counseling contexts. A person's ideological, spiritual or religious background is rarely addressed, or there is uncertainty about how to deal with it.

Religion and spirituality can have a supportive function and be an element of healing after traumatic experiences. They can provide a sense of belonging, strengthen resilience, and place an event in a larger context of meaning. However, experiences in a religious community or spiritual movement can also be the cause of trauma and a major stressor. Ideas such as "negative energies", sin, guilt, curse, hell, demons, etc. can have a strong effect, even if they are never addressed in therapy or counseling. Even less religious people are not free of superstitions. Many use good luck charms and talismans, or avoid imagining a future event positively for fear of thereby "tempting fate," or knock on wood to avert it (imagining worst-case scenarios, on the other hand, seems okay).

Spirituality in the field of psychotherapy and psychological counseling often falls into two extremes: either the field is completely ignored and never comes up, or at the other extreme, therapy itself is turned into a spiritual experience, a healing ritual. As a result, many services are offered that attempt to supplement counseling and therapy with pastoral care, shamanism, elements of esotericism, or other spiritual concepts.

My psychotherapist said he would use an additional diagnostic tool, and for that he would need my date and time of birth. He then presented me with a chart that identified me as a "projector." In further treatment, he kept referring to it, saying that my type would never allow me to take the initiative and that I should concentrate on

---

[3] The Gretchen question is an uncomfortable question that gets right to the heart of a problem. It comes from Johann Wolfgang von Goethe's "Faust I" and was originally addressed by Margarethe to Dr. Faust.

waiting and reacting. The whole thing was a little scary to me, but I trusted him; after all, he was the psychotherapist. I thought, he'll know what he's doing. But I felt less and less understood and had the impression that he really wanted to squeeze me into this scheme, and I thus had even less leeway than before. Then I inquired what this diagnostic system actually is and I was blindsided: It is pure esotericism.

Faith can be a strong source of power, but it can also be easily abused to manipulate and exercise control. Now, alternative treatment concepts and spiritual approaches are increasingly finding their way into therapeutic work. Shamanic rituals, regression, astrology, energetics, morphological fields and many more are very popular with some therapists and clients. Jessica Schab, who has experienced guru worship firsthand, talks about how easy it is to fall from one faith addiction to another. As an example, she cites Alcoholics Anonymous, who try to replace addiction with faith in God. Psychotherapy must not offer a definitive truth and thus dependence on the counselor as a possible solution.

In Austria, psychotherapy is a legally regulated health profession with the obligation to use only scientifically recognized methods. The Ministry of Health has written a guideline that demands a strict demarcation from esoteric, spiritual and religious methods [13]:

Psychotherapeutic education, training, and continuing education shall [...] *refrain from offering any kind of esoteric content, spiritual rituals and religious teachings of salvation without exception.* [...].

Psychotherapy is not able to give generally binding answers in the sense of "truths" to existential questions or even a transcendent reality, nor can it answer questions of values and meaning. Thus, serious psychotherapists will not propagate universally valid models, but will rather search together with their patients for individual solution possibilities (among other things, if necessary, also for questions of values and meaning). [...].

Cult-like groups in the surrounding field of esotericism, spirituality, fundamentalism, "shamanism" and/or "neoshamanism" or religion can incapacitate the individual, separate relationships, paint in "black-and-white", indoctrinate with teachings often alien to reality and financially exploit the followers. This clearly shows the difference between scientifically based psychotherapeutic methods, which aim at psychological recovery, and practices based on beliefs.

An apt and necessary distinction. However, the fierce controversies surrounding this guideline show how differently Austrian psychotherapists evaluate this issue.

In Germany, there are different rights and regulations for the practice of psychotherapy, depending on the professional group. Medical, psychological and child and youth psychotherapists are only allowed to use scientifically recognized therapy methods with proven effectiveness. They must also have a degree in medicine, psychology, education or social pedagogy. In the future, these different training paths for psychotherapists will be replaced by a uniform 5-year psychotherapy course. The professional title will then only be psychotherapist; the first courses of study were established in 2020 [14]. Heilpraktiker are allowed to use psychotherapy, but are not allowed to call themselves psychotherapists. They are allowed to use all therapeutic methods without proven training – regardless of whether they are scientifically recognized or not. The training of these non-medical practitioners is generally not regulated by the state. For the license as Heilpraktiker limited to the field of psychotherapy the same regulations apply with the restriction that only psychological and no physical ailments may be treated [15].

It is advisable to ask for the guidelines and concepts on which the treatment is based when you seek therapy, psychological counseling or supervision. Sometimes the ideological foundation of a person can be guessed from the homepage, sometimes you experience surprises. If it seems important to you that the person represents a certain attitude, or if you want to avoid coming into contact with esoteric concepts, bring this up right away in the initial interview or during the first contact: *"In order for you and I to be a good match, I need to make sure you don't pull out the divining rod, invoke the "knowing field," or do an exorcism with my ancestors."*

Psychologists, therapists, coaches, counselors should first reflect on their own attitude towards spirituality and become aware of their own experiences, values and judgments.

My personal relationship to religion/spirituality [16]:

- How was religion dealt with in my family?
- What does my religiosity/spirituality look like today?
- Why am I (still/no longer) a member of a church/religious community? Do I openly advocate my religiosity or atheism? In which contexts do I want to talk about it, in which not?
- How does my own spirituality (atheism, agnosticism) and my own value system impact my work with clients?
- How do I deal with clients' faith constructs?
- How do I deal with clients who grant me guru status? How do I prevent myself from adopting this flattering position? Who is my supervisor; where do I get feedback when I start to become too vain and self-important? How do I provide healthy (self-) criticism?

In the treatment of psychological conditions, as with physical conditions, it is important to reflect on the individual explanations of the illness held by the client. The eight questions according to Arthur Kleinman are also applicable here.

The beliefs of the clients and their attitude towards essential issues of life may be given space in a therapy and counseling process. The questions should be asked much more often, but the answers must be discovered autonomously by the client:

- Who or what gives you support in difficult situations?
- Do you believe in God, gods, divine powers?
- Is there a meaning behind suffering, illness and death?
- Who influences your life? Are there supernatural influences? Do they have a positive or negative effect? Can these forces be influenced by you? Is there a destiny? Is there chance, or is everything in life predetermined, directed by external forces? How great do you estimate the scope of your own will?
- Is there justice? If yes: In what way does it become effective? If no: What consequence does this have for you and the world in which you live?
- What do the concepts of guilt and atonement mean to you?
- What concepts of faith were held in your family of origin? Which ones have you retained, and which ones have you broken away from?
- Are there any positive or negative experiences with spirituality/religion?
- Do you know the longing to have a spiritual experience?
- What gives you hope?
- In what moments do you feel a sense of belonging?
- Would you describe yourself as superstitious? In what life situations?
- What influence was/is there from other people's religiosity? Are there parallels and differences with your life partner?
- Are you afraid of death? How do you deal with it?
- What are your ideas about death? Is there an afterlife? What does it look like and who has access to it? If there is no further existence after death, what are the consequences for your life? What does the subject of mortality trigger in you?
- Do you sometimes wonder about the meaning of life? What gives your life meaning? What goal does it lead to? How do you measure, in concrete terms, the meaningfulness of your existence?

As in medicine, there are also treatment methods and concepts in psychology, psychotherapy, coaching and social counseling that are not evidence-based and are partly based on dubious sources. It is even more difficult in this field to distinguish reputable from dubious providers. Family constellations, for example, can be used seriously as a proven technique from the spectrum of methods of systemic family therapy, but they can also be misused for a kind of family voodoo, in which allegedly the spirits of the ancestors take possession of the performers and baseless allegations about the persons are postulated. The training of the constellation leader is not automatically a guarantee for a serious application. It makes sense to ask the facilitator about the concepts of effectiveness on which his work is based before signing up for a weekend seminar or therapeutic accompaniment: How does it work? Where did you receive your training? What role models do you refer to? What is the therapeutic effect? Who determines the truth content? Is there a pre-treatment and an aftercare?

> *It cannot be that therapists offer methods that do not reduce the suffering of those affected, but in some cases even increase it. Especially a therapist is obliged to ask himself/herself if he/she works properly and helps instead of harming.* (Lydia Benecke, criminal psychologist)

How do I recognize serious providers in psychology/psychotherapy/counseling/coaching?

- How sound is the training? Terms such as coaching, family constellation, psychological counseling are not protected by law, anyone can use them without the appropriate qualification. Does the person have a serious education and professional experience in this field? If there is little evidence of a person's background on the homepage, caution is advised. Claims such as "has accompanied many successful change processes for years", "has been researching alternative healing methods for decades" are worthless without evidence. Also terms like institute, university, research institution … can be an empty facade. Titles are also no guarantee of competence, and conspicuously many pompous-sounding titles are rather a warning sign.
- What methods are used? Can the mechanism of action, the theory behind the method be explained in a comprehensible way? How reputable and well-known is the method? Can the provider give you literature about it? What feedback on the method do you receive from the respective professional association, on Internet sites such as Psiram, or from cult counseling centers?
- Is it claimed that with this method EVERYONE can manage to solve ALL problems quickly and forever? [17]

- Are the costs/prices in the comparable average and is an invoice issued? Beware of "energy compensation", payment on a donation basis, unspecified success fees! Absolutely unserious is an offer if you are urged to sign and pay as soon as possible and the payment is supposed to have an effect on your problem. *"The money is an impulse to the universe and shows that you are serious, and thus the treatment starts to work from the deposit."*

The coach told me to deposit the whole amount immediately, then it is already an impulse in the cosmos, and thus the treatment starts to work immediately. If I hesitate, my mind-ego will take over and prevent my development. My heart knows that this course is good for me, and I want to listen more to my heart. He justified the high cost of 30,000 euros for coaching for one year by saying that higher costs would also result in higher motivation and that my blockages to success would dissolve. Then I could recoup these costs effortlessly; he had already observed this with many of his protégés.

- Are you urged and guided to recruit other people for the course/offer? Are there success bonuses for this, do appointments take place to which you are to invite your friends and family and which have a clear advertising character for the system?
- Is there a treatment contract? Are you pressured to sign quickly? Are there dependencies, and are you required to perform work? *"We had to wash the therapist's car, clean his house and take care of his garden. He called that seva yoga. It was important to reach enlightenment, he said, and would help let go of our egos."*
- Are there any confidentiality clauses that prohibit you from sharing course content with others? Are rituals, events, one-on-one sessions a secret that you must keep? This does not apply to personal statements from other participants, which are often kept confidential; it is suspicious if you have to maintain silence about content and procedures.
- If you want to quit early, are you pressured to stay? Are you threatened with negative spiritual/psychological consequences? *"If you leave, you will hurt the energetic field of the group and jeopardize the success of others."*
- One of the best clues as to whether you are being subjected to a cult-like structure that serves the interests of the provider rather than your development is to ask: How does the provider respond to criticism? Is it used and encouraged as a constructive contribution to improvement and development, or is it blanketly rejected, perceived as an attack, and interpreted as a flaw of the person criticizing? *"My criticism was an expression of my ego, I had to let it go completely, only in this way was spiritual development possible."*

"I was told that my doubts did not come from myself at all, but were whispered to me by Satan. There was only one way to deal with demonic attacks of this kind: pray and ignore." "That I would even ask these questions was a sign of my spiritual immaturity. He said I should wait and see, then in the later course levels everything would make sense."

- How are other fields of the health care system, other methods of treatment talked about? Are visits to the doctor and taking medication discouraged? Are enemy stereotypes cultivated, are black-and-white portrayals common? Does the provider see themselves as the only source of healing far superior to all others?

- As time goes on, do you feel more and more the need to have the senior person sign off on every decision? Do you rely more and more on his/her judgment rather than your own? Does the person actively encourage this as well?

If you suspect you are being improperly cared for, seek further opinions and treatment recommendations, as is already common in medicine. If the treatment seems frivolous and harmful to you, contact health authorities, professional associations, cult counseling centers, business representatives and consumer protection associations. Legally, the situation is even more difficult than in the medical field when it comes to claiming compensation for damages and removing dangerous offers from circulation. But with every complaint, you raise awareness of this problem. Unfortunately, problematic providers are still far too rarely held accountable and therefore act with great self-confidence.

Takeaway

In the field of psychology, psychotherapy, counseling and coaching, dubious and even harmful concepts and treatment methods can be found, which are often difficult to distinguish from legitimate ones. The number of problematic providers is particularly high in this field. Consumers should pay attention to the following points: Soundness of the training of the provider and the method, professional framework, no unrealistic promises, no guru airs, no attempts to manipulate you with emotional blackmail, no imposition of supernatural elements, cooperation with other disciplines, constructive handling of criticism.

> **Food for Thought**
>
> Have you yourself had experiences with particularly good or particularly bad medical and psychological care? What were the decisive factors in each case? How would you like to be treated as a patient?
>   What makes you trust the person treating you? Where do you get information when you fall ill? Have you ever reviewed a form of treatment? In what way?

10.3   Social and Youth Work

Counteracting radicalization processes, supporting critical thinking, providing access to education and science, and protecting clients from exploitation are also central concerns of social and youth work.

Andreas Peham works at the Documentation Center of Austrian Resistance (DÖW), the most important research institution on right-wing extremism in Austria, and also works with school classes on extremism and conspiracy myths. He sees a tendency towards extremism among young people who were unable to build up a sense of basic trust at home, grew up with a lot of violence in an emotionally unstable environment, and as a result exhibit an inner emotional neediness. There is also an increased readiness to develop distrust and doubt toward state institutions and mainstream media:

> *Conspiracy theory has a counterphobic effect, existential fear is banished by transforming it into a concrete fear. In addition, there is the narcissistic benefit, the increase of power in the pseudo-competence.*

In the discussion, he is primarily concerned not with imparting knowledge, but with building relationships:

> *I don't get involved at all about the particular conspiracy theory, I don't try to refute it, because experience shows that doesn't help. I just say that I don't believe it, and then try to talk about where such conspiracy theories come from. I label them as superstition, myth, but don't dwell on them for long.*

He sees focusing on their resources rather than deficits as an important attitude in working with young people:

> *I find skepticism about a media-mediated world fundamentally positive. I just try to show other ways to encourage discussions among each other, to point out contradic-*

tions and to ask the question that is wrongly answered in the conspiracy myth: What are the interests behind it?

An example: In a workshop Muslim youths introduced the conspiracy myth that the terrorist organization "Islamic State" (IS) does not exist at all and is only a fake invented by Americans to harm Muslims. The attraction of this myth, and at the same time a resource worth connecting to, is the young people's desire as Muslims not to be equated with terrorists. Their experience is that after every attack, hostility against Muslims increases, and they do not understand why a certain group of fanatical Muslims can have an interest in this. The following discussion focuses on the question: *"Who benefits from this hostility?"* One answer might be that when anti-Muslim hostility is high, there are more comrades-in-arms to be recruited for jihad. IS thus has an interest in this enmity because it improves recruitment conditions. In this way, skepticism and critical questioning can also be directed against the conspiracy myth itself and thus become a constructive resource.

For social worker Fabian Reicher, too, the focus is on the relationship. As an employee of the Austrian Extremism Information Centre, his work focuses on prevention and exit work with radicalized and at-risk youth. He likes to use biographical narrative conversation techniques [18]. Here, the focus moves away from the argumentative-judgmental attempt to convince to telling a person's story: "How did you come to this attitude? How did you become the person you are today?" In this approach, you work a lot with your own values, ideas, questions, uncertainties, difficulties, with your own biography. Authenticity is important and also offering yourself as a role model. Young people find it cool to talk to an adult who is interested in them and also reveals something about themselves.

A selection of interventions that can be used [19]:

- **Recognition approach:** perceiving youth as experts in their life world, acknowledging their skills and resources, and granting them competence in developing and changing values and ideologies.
- **Empathic approach:** Showing empathy for the needs and personal experiences of young people, for experiences of discrimination, exclusion and powerlessness. At the same time, it is important to foster a connection to the needs of others and, through the change of perspective, also to awaken empathy for victims of inhuman and discriminatory ideologies and actions.
- **Mirroring approach:** Reflect on the (emotional) effect of what is said on oneself and on third parties. How do I feel when I hear this? How would

your girlfriend, your mother react? How would my gay friend feel when he hears this insult?

- **Relation to everyday life:** What are the consequences of this attitude in everyday life? In what ways can/should it be lived out in everyday life? What harm can it do to the person, for example, through criminal consequences or through the reactions of the environment?
- **Uncertainty approach:** Questioning the worldview presented, drawing attention to contradictions. Often only ideological fragments are adopted, there is a lot of half-knowledge. Think the slogans through to the end: *"The so-called great replacement that the Identitarians like to cite: What does that mean in concrete terms? How would we stop ethnopluralism? Deportation? Executions?"*
- **Parallelization approach:** Extremist ideologies use similar mechanisms and have comparable goals and methods. Highlight these parallels and make the intent behind them clear.
- **Reframing approach:** ideological elements are reinterpreted through a different way of looking at them. Alternative framing can give the content a surprising, more constructive meaning. *"The great jihad is about fighting the devil within you. That's an important theme, fighting the devil within yourself."*
- **Concrete utopia:** What would a perfect world look like? What would be the first steps in that direction? Concrete joint action helps to overcome the feeling of powerlessness and promotes the experience of self-efficacy.

Fabian Reicher describes the concrete implementation like this:

In youth work, the most important tool is oneself, one's own values and attitudes. It's about giving the kids feedback in the protective space of the relationship: How does it come across when you say that? There's no relationship breakup, no matter what they say. They can try it out and learn. If it gets to be too much for me, I'll slam a door and tell them I've had enough, that if I didn't know them, I'd think they were total Nazis now or be afraid of them. They are not told enough about how their behavior is received by others. They want feedback when they show an extreme position. It is also important to teach them that being a Nazi or having extreme positions is not pleasant. I have to provide content for the learning field, I can't leave it apolitical, I have to take a position in conversations. In group settings, I have to intervene immediately if there are homophobic statements, for example. It may be that there are gay or lesbian young people in the group, so I have to convey to all of them that such a statement is not normal and not okay and will not be left unchallenged. And they have to experience that they cannot make such a statement without being contradicted, and that I am absolutely not cool with it. That's very important, otherwise it becomes normalized. Contradiction is always important when someone is dehumanized! After that, start narratively: How do you come up with this?

It can also be helpful to look for allies in the peer group and to involve people who are relevant to the scene, for example, members who set the tone in the fan clubs of large soccer teams. As a social worker, Reicher uses his opportunities to provide people with concrete support for their problems; in the long term, this enables him to build up a good reputation in the community. This has been particularly successful with the online project Jamal al-Khatib [20]: Here, former jihadists and young people who had considered leaving for Syria wrote texts that were then turned into videos. In a comprehensive online campaign [21], the subject areas otherwise occupied by the jihadists were filled with their own content. One goal here is to soften extreme positions. When it comes to wearing headscarves, for example, there seem to be only two positions in the discussion: the headscarf as a sign of oppression or as a duty. The online campaign aims to mediate positions in between, to question fundamentalism, but to address the issues of young people. Extremists have an identitarian and exclusivist framing that aims at powerlessness and alienation rather than empowerment. One example is the campaign "Uyghurs, We Don't Forget You!" [22] The framing of the Salafists is: *"The world is looking the other way because it's only Muslims."* Being Muslim is the identity-building component; a sense of powerlessness is created. Only we Salafists help. The Jamal al-Khatib campaigns convey: The issue concerns us all! What can we all do about it?

We pick up on the anger, don't appease, but differentiate more; for example, we have a video of an Orthodox Jew who discusses the problem. This shows that this is an issue that not only Muslims are interested in. And we offer low-threshold activities to get involved, to feel empowerment, e.g. a sticker challenge and the possibility to share info online and show solidarity. We occupy the topics that extremists otherwise occupy and give them a spin in the direction of inclusion, empowerment, away from the victim attitude into a solidarity attitude. We actively determine the discourse, our videos were also shared by many Salafist sites. What was important was that we let those affected have their say directly and made calls to action. (Fabian Reicher)

With NISA [23], a platform was created by girls and young women, that deals specifically with patriarchal structures and counters them with alternative narratives.

Both experts, Andreas Peham and Fabian Reicher, emphasize the importance of not neglecting social roots of radicalization and not focusing solely on individual biographical causes. In order to combat extremist and divisive tendencies in society, the focus must not only be on the individual, but also on how extremist tendencies can be countered in society as a whole [24]. When people experience exclusion and perceive the social and political system as unjust, mistrust in decision-makers and state institutions increases. This prepares the breeding ground for conspiracy myths, segregation and radicalization.

> **Takeaway**
>
> Radicalization is a multi-layered process that cannot be countered with bans or information alone. On the one hand, it is important to set clear limits to inhumane statements and actions, but to perceive the acting person in his or her history, motives and needs and to reach out by building an appreciative relationship. Empathy, a focus on a person's resources and measures that strengthen autonomy and the experience of self-efficacy help to question extremist ideologies that create identity.

References

1. Blog "Stiftung Gurutest". https://www.derstandard.at/story/2000109455158/wie-viel-nazi-ideologie-steckt-im-begriff-schulmedizin. Accessed on: 11. Febr. 2021
2. Hirschhausen E (2016) Wunder wirken Wunder. Wie Medizin und Magie und heilen. Rowohlt, Reinbek
3. Ernst E (2021) Heilung oder Humbug? 150 alternativmedizinische Verfahren von Akupunktur bis Yoga. Springer, Berlin, p 54
4. Burnett D (2016) The idiot brain. A neuroscientist explains what your head is really up to. Guardian, Faber & Faber, London
5. http://witze.net/medizinstudenten-witze. Accessed on: 11. Febr. 2021
6. medizin transparent (2021) Checkliste Gesundheitsmythen – Fake news erkennen. https://www.medizin-transparent.at/ueber/gesundheitsmythen-fake-news-erkennen. Accessed on: 7. Febr. 2021
7. Humanistischer Pressedienst. https://hpd.de/artikel/tod-einer-13-jaehrigen-durch-naives-gottvertrauen-17718. Accessed on: 9. Febr. 2021
8. Jehovas Zeugen (2021) Warum akzeptieren Jehovas Zeugen keine Bluttransfusionen? https://www.jw.org/de/jehovas-zeugen/oft-gefragt/jehovas-zeugen-warum-keine-bluttransfusion/. Accessed on: 11. Febr. 2021. Der Oberste Gerichtshof (2012) Verweigerung einer medizinisch indizierten lebensrettenden Bluttransfusion durch Zeugin Jehovas verstößt gegen die Schadensminderungspflicht. https://www.ogh.gv.at/entscheidungen/entscheidungen-ogh/verweigerung-einer-medizinisch-

indizierten-lebensrettenden-bluttransfusion-durch-zeugin-jehovas-verstoesst-gegen-die-schadensminderungspflicht/. Accessed on: 11. Febr. 2021

9. Broschüre "Glaubensfreiheit versus Kindeswohl". https://sekten-info-nrw.de/information/infomaterial

10. Meiss O (2009) Kontext und Wirkung von Suggestionen. In: Revenstorf D, Peter B (eds) Hypnose in Psychotherapie, Psychosomatik und Medizin. Springer, Heidelberg, pp 92–103

11. Bejenke C (2009) Vorbereitung auf medizinische Eingriffe. In: Revenstorf D, Peter B (eds) Hypnose in Psychotherapie, Psychosomatik und Medizin. Springer, Heidelberg, pp 630–640

12. Dabney E (2011) 101 Dinge, die ich gern gewusst hätte, als ich anfing, mit Hypnose zu arbeiten. Carl-Auer, Heidelberg

13. Richtlinie zur Frage der Abgrenzung der Psychotherapie von esoterischen, spirituellen, religiösen und weltanschaulichen Angeboten sowie Hinweise für PatientInnen bzw. KlientInnen. https://www.sozialministerium.at/dam/jcr:14f29365-606a-41d5-84eb-a5f7a6e142ed/Abgrenzung_der_Psychotherapie_von_esotereischen,_spirituellen,_religiösen_und_weltanschaulichen_Angeboten_sowie_Hinweise_für_PatientInnen_bzw._KlientI.pdf. Accessed on: 11. Febr. 2021

14. Bundesministerium für Gesundheit: Moderne Ausbildung für Psychotherapeutinnen und Psychotherapeuten. https://www.bundesgesundheitsministerium.de/psychotherapeutenausbildung.html. Accessed on: 11. Febr. 2021

15. Berufsverband Psychosoziale Berufe: Psychotherapie und Heilpraktikerzulassung. https://www.dgvt-bv.de/news-details/?tx_ttnews%5Btt_news%5D=321&cHash=dbde646daa5dd7a56129aef1579842c0. Accessed on: 3. Mai 2021

16. Based on seminar handouts by German Müller and Sylvia Neuberger

17. Dierbach H (2009) Die Seelenpfuscher: Pseudotherapien, die krank machen. Rowohlt, Reinbek bei Hamburg

18. Neuburg F, Kühne S, Reicher F (2020) Soziale Netzwerke und Virtuelle Räume: Aufsuchendes Arbeiten zwischen analogen und digitalen Welten. In: Diebäcker M, Wild G (eds) Streetwork und Aufsuchende Soziale Arbeit im öffentlichen Raum. Springer, Wiesbaden, pp 167–184

19. Lippe F, Reidinger V (2019) Begleitende Praxisforschung: Jamal al-Khatib – Mein Weg! und NISA x Jana. https://a596b1ed-e408-443e-99d4-c7960d4ae3a1.filesusr.com/ugd/0cc6d7_74abbd599932401ea6d47457a3859758.pdf. Accessed on: 23. Febr. 2021

20. YouTube-Kanal Jamal al-Khatib. https://www.youtube.com/channel/UCKmWuKvMLGHQ4Z0VaVjwYVQ, https://www.facebook.com/jamalalkhatibmeinweg/. Accessed on: 6. Febr. 2021

21. Reicher F, Lippe F (2019) Jamal al-Khatib – Mein Weg! Online-Campaigning als Methode der Politischen Bildung. https://www.e-beratungsjournal.net/wp-content/uploads/2019/05/reicher_lippe.pdf. Accessed on: 6. Febr. 2021

22. Jugendarbeit Wien. #UIGUREN #WIR VERGESSEN EUCH NICHT! Eine Kampagne von Jamal al-Khatib. https://www.jugendarbeit.wien/uiguren-wir-vergessen-euch-nicht-eine-kampagne-von-jamal-al-khatib/. Accessed on: 6. Febr. 2021

23. YouTube-Kanal NISA. https://www.youtube.com/channel/UC702G0F82JOV VQ4zPHR3RtA. Accessed on: 6. Febr. 2021

24. Reicher F (2015) Deradikalisierung und Extremismusprävention im Jugendalter. Eine kritische Analyse. Erschienen in: soziales_kapital, wissenschaftliches journal österreichischer fachhochschul-studiengänge soziale arbeit Nr. 14 (2015). Rubrik "Junge Wissenschaft". Standort Wien

Part III

Practical Tips

We have covered the most important situations in which discussions of irrational ideas can occur in Part II. Much of this can be transferred in part to similarly situated contexts, for example from the family to the closer circle of friends. However, there are of course also things that are regularly repeated in such discussions, regardless of the context. These include, for example, sentences that one hears again and again, arguments and pseudo-arguments that crop up regularly, which are difficult to answer at first glance, but which hardly stand up to critical scrutiny. To this end, we first look at the substantive validity of these statements, but also ask how they can be reasonably countered. Finally, beyond the individual situations, there are also principles and practical tips that are worth keeping in mind in general.

11

Sentences You Hear Again and Again

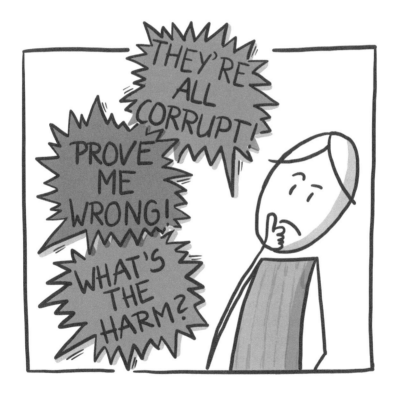

H. G. Hümmler, U. Schiesser, *Fact and Prejudice*,
https://doi.org/10.1007/978-3-662-66032-4_11

Anyone who regularly engages in discussions with believers as a scientifically minded person will at some point develop a tendency to roll his eyes at certain statements: There are phrases that one encounters again and again because they enjoy unshakable popularity among believers of different persuasions. They often do so because they are difficult to answer, even if they generally do not really present valid arguments.

11.1 He Who Heals Is Right

The favorite mantra of alternative medicine practitioners is actually a truism. The devil is in the implied claim that the occurrence of an improvement should prove that someone has been healed. In fact, in the vast majority of diseases, at least a temporary improvement occurs at some point on its own. A person who happens to have just performed a rain dance at that time cannot claim to have cured the patient. The same applies if this rain dance took place in close temporal connection with a serious medical therapy, which could also have caused the improvement.

Proving that an intervention has actually had a relevant positive or negative influence on the course of health is the biggest problem of medical research. Reports on individual cases simply do not contribute anything to this, and even careful follow-up observations on a large number of patients or epidemiological analyses on an entire population have only very limited probative value because of the confounding factors that are difficult to control. In order to arrive at reasonably reliable conclusions about a therapy method, the course of treatment in treated and untreated test subjects must be compared in a so-called intervention study. For this purpose, both groups must be as comparable as possible and ideally randomized. The non-treated subjects must receive a substitute that is as identical as possible to the actual treatment, except for the factor to be investigated. This substitute is called a placebo – so it is not necessarily the sugar pills often associated with this term. Finally, until the results are evaluated, neither the subjects nor the treating and investigating staff should know who belongs to the treated and who to the control group (double blinding). At the same time, these high requirements limit the number of test subjects, because one does not want to deprive sick people of a recognizably effective therapy or expose them to a possibly harmful treatment. As a consequence, only an expert review of all available studies on a topic in evidence based medicine (which, unfortunately, is often literally translated to German)[1] can be a statement about the effectiveness of a medical intervention. The possibly completely honest impression of individual doctors, alternative practitioners or spiritual healers that they have healed someone says absolutely nothing about their actual success. To let oneself be blinded by such subjective experiences is not uncommon even among seriously trained physicians, as Florian Albrecht, a family doctor who used to be open to alternative methods himself, reports from discussions with colleagues:

> *They will always say: But I have had other experiences. And again and again experiences are placed above scientific data.*

The former homeopathic physician Natalie Grams recognizes herself in this:

> *I really believe that for me, as for many other people, it was because of these positive experiences. It helped me, so it must be true. If someone had told me earlier how little you can rely on the individual experience in medicine, I might have had doubts sooner.*

The same applies to the claim, often presented as justification for implausible alternative medical methods, that they activate self-healing powers or strengthen the immune system (which, given the dangerous nature of some autoimmune diseases, would also be less than desirable). Both would have to be proven in studies according to the standards just described. However, the healers in question usually fail to provide this proof.

The only realistic answer to "He who heals is right" is the question of proof for the claimed healing success. This proof would also have to clearly distinguish the claimed success from the success of other measures, from a natural improvement or from pure coincidence.

If, however, the validity of the principles of evidence-based medicine is questioned and instead reference is made to so-called experiential knowledge, then all that remains for the substantive discussion is to point out that this form of experience is a pure belief system. It is subject to all the mechanisms of self-deception described in Chap. 2, and in a discussion it can only be countered as a belief system.

---

[1] *Evidenz* in German means the obvious or the appearance; evidence, however, means proof. If the results of science-based medicine were really evident, one could save many of the discussions considered here.

11.2 Take Something Natural First!

That substances must be healthy or at least harmless or environmentally friendly if they are of natural origin is repeated so often in public and so rarely questioned that it has become a self-evident truth for many people. Patients want, and doctors and pharmacists recommend, in many cases first of all "something herbal" if a synthetic drug does not seem absolutely necessary.

Why do we actually assume this? One of the most toxic substances we can realistically encounter in our lives, botulinum toxin (Botox), is naturally produced by bacteria in spoiled meat and was a common cause of fatal poisoning until the introduction of industrially produced nitrite curing salt. Similarly deadly is tetanospasmin, the toxin of the tetanus bacterium, whose spores are somewhere in the soil waiting to get into the wound of an injured animal (or human, for that matter). Certain jellyfish, snakes, spiders or snails contain enough venom per animal to kill several people. That new deadly pathogens arise in nature without human intervention seems so implausible to us that ever new conspiracy myths continue to swirl around the appearance of HIV and SARS-CoV-2.

There is a small kernel of rationality in this reasoning, much like the "tried and true" home remedies: We can at least expect substances that have been part of our food, our household medicine, or our daily interactions for centuries not to kill us in the short term in everyday amounts. However, it does not follow from this, for example, that they do not show harmful effects in the long term in view of the greatly increased life expectancy and cannot be carcinogenic, for example, as is the case with acrylamide, which is formed during baking, frying or grilling of completely everyday, natural foods.

Ultimately, "natural" or "proven" substances are simply more familiar to us than synthetic or even genetically engineered alternatives. Yet – partly precisely because of this very "natural" distrust of the "unnatural" – the technically developed products are usually far better examined for possible harmful effects than the natural products that are so tried and trusted. If the natural products are actually examined more closely, they often perform poorly. This is not only true of pharmaceuticals, where the poison of foxglove (digitalis) has largely become obsolete as a heart medicine, just as cod liver oil has become obsolete as a dietary supplement, and where supposedly immune-stimulating agents such as echinacea have turned out to be useless. Even in beverages, the cumarin-containing woodruff has been practically completely replaced by synthetic flavorings that taste only vaguely similar.

For me (Holm Gero Hümmler), the change in thinking during my studies came about as a result of a remark made by a fellow biology student who was actually rather a friend of nature:

If I need a medicinal active ingredient, then I want to have this one substance in a constant dosage and residue-free from a monitored production and not in a composition that changes depending on the weather with some plant residues whose effect no one knows.

This cocktail of different ingredients in herbal medicines can lead to problems not only directly, which is still relatively easy to verify, but especially in interaction with other medicines. For example, St. John's wort, which is popular against depression, interferes with the absorption of various drugs and can, for example, impair the effect of hormonal contraceptives and thus lead to unplanned pregnancies.

In Germany, the significantly reduced requirement for the safety and efficacy of herbal medicines is even expressly enshrined in law. Herbal medicines, like other medicines, can be approved on the basis of controlled studies according to the rules of evidence-based medicine – but they do not have to be. They can also, like anthroposophic or homeopathic remedies, be approved according to the so-called internal consensus, i.e. according to highly simplified rules that are only recognized within the respective field. In contrast to many anthroposophic and the vast majority of homeopathic remedies, however, herbal medicines are not placebos that are largely or completely free of active ingredients. They actually contain active substances and many other substances more, the effects of which do not even have to be researched in detail according to the law. The physician Florian Albrecht, who turned away from alternative medicine, also stresses that in medicinal herbs from ominous sources in India or China again and again poisonous substances are found in sometimes dangerous quantity. Especially in Ayurvedic "medicine" heavy metals such as lead and mercury can occur not only as unintentional contamination, but even as deliberate but not always declared additives [1].

The idea of doing something good for oneself with organic foods is also based on the erroneous conclusion that natural products must necessarily be healthy. In fact, ideally, they may contain fewer residues of synthetic pesticides. However, the effects of these residues, which are minimal in any case, on humans are generally far better studied than natural components of our cultivated plants that occur in similar quantities. In addition, there are sometimes dangerous contaminants that today actually only occur as a result of organic cultivation. The alkaloids of the ergot fungus, which attacks cereals and regularly led to mass poisoning in the Middle Ages, played practically no role in foods in the 1980s. In the meantime, recalls have been issued time and again due to contamination with ergot alkaloids, especially in cereals and flour from organic farming [2]. Tropane alkaloids, which occur in weeds such as datura and henbane, have also largely disappeared from our diet. On organic fields and subsequently around them, these poisonous plants are much more difficult to control. Here, there are repeatedly not only product recalls, but also acute cases of poisoning [3]. Poppy and buckwheat are particularly affected, but also millet, which is popular in baby food, because their small grains are very difficult to separate in the mill from the similarly large and heavy seeds of the poisonous plants.

One could write one's own books about the various advantages and disadvantages of organic farming for the environment.

Anyone who brings up these issues will quickly encounter incomprehension, disbelief and reflexive rejection, and not only from esoteric or particularly nature-loving contemporaries. It is therefore advisable not to blow up the conversation with a provocative tirade against the nature faith in general, but to underline first individual, well provable aspects and to supply further points afterwards only if there is serious interest.

11.3 Why Don't You Try It, It Won't Do Any Harm?

The reference to the supposed harmlessness of "natural" or "proven" methods is not only found in alternative medicine, but there it is particularly alarming. The ear, nose and throat specialist and homeopathy critic Christian Lübbers summarizes the risks of supposedly harmless sham therapies:

> The dangers of placebo therapy are point 1, that an effective therapy is delayed, point 2, that an effective therapy or prevention is omitted – many homeopathy believers unfortunately also refrain from effective vaccinations – and point 3, the danger of general disbelief in science.

However, there are other problem areas that are not unique to alternative medicine: The self-efficacy initially gained with the use of esoteric concepts[2] has the flip side that for the sooner or later inevitable failure of such approaches

---

[2] In psychology, self-efficacy is the conviction that one can shape one's own life and master difficult situations oneself.

always the user himself is made responsible. Having already given up suppos-edly insignificant freedoms by aligning his life with astrology, spreading con-spiracy myths or constantly carrying around sugar pills, he is also blamed for the fact that these concepts have not helped him. Thomas F., a pediatrician who used to believe in homeopathy, reports on his experiences:

> *Then always comes this reversal of guilt, then you as a patient are the ass, you used the wrong toothpaste, or black tea or coffee … you did whatever. The whole normal way of life already aggressively runs counter to homeopathy.*

In the best case, esoteric ideas about the placebo effect can actually help you get better – but you would have the placebo effect even with a treatment that has a real effect in addition. In many other cases, esoteric concepts are simply a waste of time that one finds more or less meaningful or entertaining and that can certainly provide one with support and reassurance as rituals. However, with a large part of these concepts, there is at least the potential for one to become entangled in them, to make a large part of one's life dependent on them, and to place unrealistic hopes on them. In these cases, in addition to a great deal of time, one can also lose quality of life, large amounts of money and, in the worst case, one's health.

To point out these risks at least in principle should be reasonable for a counterpart who refers to the harmlessness of certain anti-scientific concepts. If the hint proves unnecessary, because the person concerned actually only has some fun reading horoscopes in the long run, one should not do any harm. Otherwise, it may be food for thought that can be very valuable later, if the other person is in danger of giving up important freedoms or risking his health for this belief.

11.4   Quantum Physics Has Shown …

Since some years quantum physics is not only used as a proof for homeopathy, spiritual healing, charlatanry devices and other questionable healing meth-ods – it also serves as an example for a supposed "new thinking" in science, according to which "everything is connected with everything" and mind con-trols matter.

Who looks at least into the basics of actual quantum physics (for example with the book "Relative quantum nonsense – can modern physics prove eso-tericism" by author Holm Gero Hümmler – so far only available in German), will quickly find out that assertions of this kind have absolutely nothing to do with real physics. They are not new findings, but distorted images of outdated popular scientific representations and out of context, partly even freely invented, speculative statements of historical persons from the beginnings of modern physics more than 70 years ago. In fact, quantum mechanics does not say that the consciousness of the experimenter controls the result of a measurement, but on the contrary that the result of a measurement is completely random and uninfluenceable within the framework of statistical probabilities.

Those who refer to Einstein, Schrödinger or Heisenberg to justify their own theses or offers are often not at all concerned with actual findings of physics. Instead, the names of these long-dead personalities lend a semblance of authority and wisdom to statements that have turned out to be meaningless. At the same time, invoking a notoriously mathematically abstract subject like quantum physics deters critics who, in general, do not want to engage in discussions about wave equations and complex operators.

However, the vast majority of those who parrot such claims actually believe they have found a deeper insight into a new science in the platitudinous statements of those who distort Heisenberg. In such a case it can be helpful to refer to generally understandable explanations of serious physicists as a reading recommendation. Besides the (German) book and blog "Relative Quantum Nonsense", the books and blogs of the physicists Florian Aigner and Florian Freistetter as well as the (German) YouTube videos of Prof. Lemeshko are recommended. One should get involved in a discussion about details from physics only if one has the corresponding knowledge, but hints that historical quotations have only a historical meaning are actually always appropriate regarding "authorities" like Planck, Einstein, Bohr, Schrödinger or Heisenberg. After all, a large part of today's knowledge about the transition of quantum mechanical states to our "normal" world did not even exist in rudiments when Max Planck died in 1947. Heisenberg, who died later, also made his major contributions to quantum theories in the 1920s and 1930s. Serious physicists of the present, whose simplifications aimed at laymen are often taken out of context and interpreted in a distorting way, are for example the American string theorist Brian Greene or the president of the Austrian Academy of Sciences Anton Zeilinger. Likewise gladly quoted by esotericists are authors adhering to pseudo-scientific concepts like Rupert Sheldrake or Ulrich Warnke as well as physicists drifted into esotericism like Burkhard Heim, Fritjof Capra or Hans-Peter Dürr. The fact that someone is a natural scientist does not exclude that he publishes at the same time his private fantasies, which may be in conflict with a broad consensus in science.

11.5   Science Is Also Only a Belief

Behind the assertion that science is "also just a belief" or the accusation of "believing in science" there is more than just an arbitrary judgement. People who make such statements usually have a completely distorted understanding of what science actually is. When asked, they will often say that the basis of science is the memorization of textbook knowledge, which must not be questioned under any circumstances and which leads scientists to believe that they already know everything. This textbook knowledge would be created by individual outstanding personalities due to their own genius. This genius is only insufficiently grasped by the other, normal scientists because of the limitation of their horizon demanded by the system.

Sometimes "spiritual people" feel also personally close to these alleged geniuses and have the feeling to participate, on the basis of their quotations or popular science texts, directly in a wisdom which remains hidden to normal scientists in their textbooks and scientific publications. For example, ex-YouTube guru Jessica Schab reports that:

> I really believed that I understood quantum physics, that I had a deeper knowledge, when I said that everything is connected with everything.

People are also fond of quoting a sentence attributed (in this form without evidence) to Nobel Prize winner Richard Feynman: *"Anyone who thinks he has understood quantum mechanics has not understood it."*[3] This quote is especially popular with people who have not understood even the most basic concepts and equations of quantum mechanics.

This portrayal of esotericists' view of science may sound exaggerated, caricatured or polemical, but it can be found very similarly again and again in esoteric texts, which dismiss the work of today's physicists as outdated and mechanistic and instead spin a "new physics" out of anachronistic quotations of actually or supposedly important physicists from the past [4–6]. Very similar is the situation of modern scientific psychology, which is devalued or completely ignored, while esotericists claim to have found deep wisdom in fragments and quotations of Sigmund Freud and especially Carl Gustav Jung [7–11].

---

[3] The proven original form of the quote – *"There was a time when a newspaper said that only 12 men understood the theory of relativity. [...] On the other hand I can safely say that nobody understands quantum mechanics"* – was a whimsical interjection in one of Feynman's lectures – and an appeal to listeners not to naively picture quantum mechanical concepts.

Obviously, all this has little to do with actual science, which as a method is based on the constant questioning of all known knowledge. In such a realistic view of science, every scientific finding, i.e. that which has currently passed the systematic questioning, is inevitably an intermediate state, which will be expanded in the future and embedded in superordinate contexts, but which can also turn out to be wrong in parts. Thus, one can only be a scientist if one does not think that one knows everything, but on the contrary can accept that one will never know everything. Of course, as a scientist you have to know your field, because meaningful questioning is only possible if you understand what you want to question and know which questions have already been asked and dealt with in the past. While the role of individuals is often high-lighted in accounts of the history of science, real science is a collaborative effort in which individual actors make only tiny contributions to the overall picture: the medical study database PubMed lists more than 86,000 articles, mostly with multiple authors, on research into COVID-19 in 2020 alone. At CERN, sometimes several thousand scientists work on the development of a single experiment. Even the theory of relativity, as firmly linked as it is with the name Einstein, was anything but the achievement of a single person.

Florian Aigner, science communicator at the Vienna University of Technology, sums it up beautifully:

> Science is a network of opinions and arguments, where quite a lot of people together influence each other and where there is a huge number of facts and findings and results that have to fit together, like a huge net, where one node holds the other, so that you can call it science at all. If someone is a scientist and has an opinion, that is not science. Science is intersubjective, greater than what any one person can do. That increases the reliability, the weight of scientific knowledge extremely. Science is greater than any one of us and as such is trustworthy.

Far more similarity than with actual science has the scientific image of the esotericists with pseudo-scientific belief systems such as homeopathy or anthroposophy, in whose system the respective founders Hahnemann and Steiner are actually above any criticism.

In view of such fundamentally different ideas of what science actually is, a meaningful discussion of scientific content with a representative of such views is obviously very difficult. It is difficult to make up in adulthood for what the school has obviously failed to teach in the way of understanding science, if this is also countered by an established esoteric view of the world. Depending on the interests and open-mindedness of the counterpart, one can try to awaken an understanding for the basic ideas of actual science by referring to generally understandable presentations. Corresponding representations can be found for example in book form by Florian Aigner [12] and Lee McIntyre [13], in the form of blog articles [14] as well as entertaining [15] or very compact [16] videos.

11.6 The Scientists Are All Corrupt

"Has Monsanto bought scientists?" speculated the anti-lobbying lobby organization Transparency International in 2017 [17]. *"That's why you shouldn't believe every study"* was the headline of German public radio station WDR in 2016, claiming in the article that business companies bribe universities with large sums of money [18]. The Süddeutsche Zeitung wrote about *"The bought science"* and claimed in the article that there are "a vast amount of cooperations" of universities with the big car manufacturers; however, one looked for corresponding cooperations with organizations like Greenpeace in vain [19]. In reality, it takes less than 2 minutes of Google searching to find such research collaborations precisely with Greenpeace [20, 21]. Moreover, these organizations have an influence in science through their university groups, which does not cost them a cent. The author of the Süddeutsche article concludes with the statement that it was *"not to discredit the work of countless researchers in industry or in university collaborations with industry"* – after the article has done just that.

From the media, one could get the impression that scientists are paid by industry to manipulate results in a way that is favorable to corporate interests. The so-called third-party funding, which has grown strongly in recent times, arouses particular suspicion. It means that research at universities is funded by external sponsors on a project-by-project basis rather than from the university's own budget. This does indeed sound like bought science, but where does this money actually come from? In Germany, a declining 18% of this third-party funding still came from commercial sources in 2018. By far the largest source of third-party funding is the tax-funded German Research Foundation. In addition, there are funding and excellence programs from the federal government, the states and the European Union, as well as a small portion from foundations. Third-party funding from industry accounts for only 2.6% of total university spending [22].

Moreover, the fact that research projects are funded by companies does not mean in most cases that these companies have any interest at all in manipulating the results. In fact, companies usually want to use the results of the research they fund themselves, for example, to develop new products or optimize operations. This may lead to conflicts over what proportion of the results may be published, because companies naturally do not want to share the data they have financed themselves with their competitors. Here too, however, the main purpose of publishing research results is to test them against the criticism of other scientists and to improve them. Thus, by keeping too much secrecy, one harms oneself.

Of course, there are also cases in which companies have an interest in a certain result coming out of scientific research. In this case, the interest can rub off on the researchers, who do not want to lose their sponsors for future projects. However, science does not presuppose that individual scientists do not have their own interests when conducting research. That would simply be unrealistic, because researchers are also human beings. It is perfectly normal for scientists to want a certain result of their research because it corresponds to their own already published hypotheses, promotes their career, flatters their vanity, serves a "good cause" – or even the sponsor. The whole scientific method is intended to minimize the influence of such individual expectations of results on the knowledge gained. This is exactly why every field of research has its methods, according to which one has to check results; this is exactly why the methods and results are published according to uniform standards, and this is exactly why criticism by other scientists, some of whom will practically always have the opposite expectations, helps. Where problems have arisen in the past, for example through attempts by the tobacco industry to cast doubt on the dangers of smoking with questionable studies, the control mechanisms in the standards of science are constantly being developed. For example, when results are published, donors who might have an interest in a particular outcome of the study, as well as conceivable conflicts of interest on the part of researchers, must now be disclosed.

Where scientific results serve as the basis for decisions by authorities, legislators have in some cases created additional control mechanisms. For example, for the approval of drugs, manufacturers must submit scientific studies according to certain standards in order to prove the safety and efficacy of the drugs. Naturally, a company has an interest in ensuring that a new drug, in the development of which it has typically invested hundreds of millions of euros, may also be sold, and naturally this company would like to influence the outcome of the relevant studies in its favor. Competing companies and health insurers who have to pay for the new drugs and who also act as funders of studies, however, would like to have the opposite outcome and will, together with competing researchers, take a particularly critical look at the published results. Regulatory agencies also generally have no interest in producing scandals later by approving unnecessary products, and employ their own experts to critically review the studies. In the past, it is said to have occasionally happened that studies that were unfavorable for a company were concealed. For this reason, all studies that are later to be used for drug approval must now be registered in a publicly readable form before the study begins, with a precise description of the research question and method.

So science as a whole is quite robust against attempts to influence it by funders – not because individual scientists are not susceptible to influence, but because science has always assumed that individual scientists can be subject to all sorts of influences and interests.

However, science communicator Florian Aigner sees a clear resistance to economic influences even among individual scientists themselves:

> *In addition, some people have a distorted image of the scientist: They are all bought, they don't care about our health, they only look after their own money. The fact that people in medical research are also people who have children they want to be healthy; that people in chemical research want to have a healthy environment is not clear to most people. I know more environmentally-minded people from the chemical research field than any other field. Especially when it comes to the environment or health, people like to construct a dichotomy of technology and science on the one hand and nature on the other. This dichotomy is fiction, it does not exist. Of course there are business and corporate interests, but that is not science.*

Incidentally, it is not the case that there are no business interests in unscientific ideas: in the field of homeopathic and anthroposophic "medicines" alone, there are several manufacturers in Germany with sales in the hundreds of millions. In the past, they have not necessarily been squeamish in their dealings with critics and have, for example, tried to intimidate the homeopathy critic Natalie Grams by legal means [23] or paid bloggers to defame critics [24]. Also the marketing of individual esoteric offers as well as education and training for those who live from it, are in total a billion dollar business.

11.7 Science Is Cold and Unromantic

Old white men in lab coats, unconscionable technology lovers obsessed with universal feasibility, inventing weapons of mass destruction or genetically engineering horror creatures, loners who calculate gloomy prophecies on mountains of written notes. The image of scientists in pop culture is not necessarily a sympathetic one. Above all, science is seen as calculating, cold and unromantic. If scientists are considered to have any passion at all, it is at best in a deviant, destructive form.

For people who have dedicated their lives to science, on the other hand, such a view is often unimaginable – simply because they experience the opposite in their work. In 2019, the image of computer scientist Katie Bouman went around the world, gleeful as a child when her computer displayed the image of a black hole. It was the first ever reconstructed image of such an object, the result of years of work by Bouman's entire team with newly developed computational methods based on a vast amount of astrophysical measurement data. Astrophysicists with their research on the formation of the earth, our solar system, other celestial bodies and the universe as a whole, have the best chance to make the fascination and sometimes breathtaking beauty of their results comprehensible to outsiders.

Not only the chemists mentioned by Florian Aigner, but also many biologists are committed environmentalists and often came to their field precisely through their enthusiasm for ecological issues. Tobias Reiners, who studies the genome of European hamsters at the Senckenberg Society for Nature Research in Frankfurt, is also chairman of the Hessian Society for Ornithology and Nature Conservation. In his appearances at science slams, he fascinates audiences with an exciting detective story about the search for the reasons why his home state's hamster population has suddenly disappeared.

For people who may find science interesting, but not exciting or romantic, such science slams offer an opportunity to see mostly young scientists presenting their field of research in an engaging, understandable and funny way to an enthusiastic lay audience. After a series of short presentations, usually limited to 10 min, the audience chooses a winner.

Sometimes the beauty of a research area can only be seen after some time spent on the topic. My (Holm Gero Hümmler) view of the sky has changed permanently with the study of my minor subject meteorology:

When I started to study meteorology in my first semester, I suddenly could no longer see a sunset, but only the high particle load during air temperature inversion, which made the light of the setting sun appear even redder. But then – it must have been in my fourth semester – I saw a thunderstorm coming at some point, and now I knew about the gigantic energies that are released in such a cloud, the hailstones floating in the furious updraft, the huge static charge that is discharged when you only see a slight flash from a distance – and I thought to myself: Man, that's majestic. And I remain fascinated by every thunderstorm to this day.

Conveying this particular beauty of scientific knowledge is an important point when talking to people who reject science. *"The beauty of scientific understanding and the thrill of the chase,"* underlines British psychologist Susan Blackmore, whom this chase has turned from a believer in paranormal phenomena into a skeptic.:

> *Of course not everybody has that curiosity, which you need to have that attitude. There is this terrible idea, that, if you don't believe in all those things, that you are an unspiritual person, that you are probably a vile, unkind, cruel, terrible human being. That always shines through in those discussions; the internet is full of it. Understanding that spectacular experiences can have natural causes doesn't take away the spirituality for me. That is hard to convey, but I find it so important.*

11.8 Prove to Me that It Is Not So!

The demand for a reversal of the burden of proof is a regularly recurring part of discussions with believers. Sometimes it is demanded to prove the non-existence of ghosts or other supernatural beings, sometimes the non-existence of extraterrestrial visitors in the present or in the distant past, sometimes the impossibility of parapsychological phenomena and sometimes the ineffectiveness of so-called alternative therapies. Proofs derived from principles or from other natural sciences are thereby regularly called mechanistic, naively science-believing or dismissed (in complete misjudgement of the actual meaning of the term) as positivistic.[4] Friends of homeopathy, for example, are usually unimpressed by the realization that homeopathic high potencies contain no active ingredients at all, but only sugar. They regularly see evidence of this, for example in the form of demonstrative homeopathic overdoses, as proof of the skeptics' naïveté.

The American astronomer Carl Sagan is credited with the sentence: *"Extraordinary claims require extraordinary evidence."* According to this, the onus of proof would be on the person who makes the more extraordinary claim that deviates from the scientific consensus. Why this should be so, however, is not obvious to everyone. For some homeopaths, the efficacy of modern medicines, which is comprehensible on the level of individual chemical interactions, may seem more extraordinary than the scientifically untenable, but in a magical sense plausible, similarity principle of their own teaching. As

---

[4] Positivism was a philosophical current that demanded that science limit its scope to sensually perceptible things and assign all other aspects to other spheres not accessible to science.

an argument in a discussion with believers, then, Sagan's claim may be met with the accusation that double standards are being applied.

In fact, however, in most cases it is already impossible in principle to provide the required counter-evidence. It is true that studies conducted according to careful scientific criteria regularly fail to find evidence of an efficacy of homeopathy that goes beyond the placebo effect. However, this does not prove that there could not be at least in principle some effect of homeopathy, and such studies are not at all suitable to exclude with absolute certainty such an effect of homeopathic remedies, which is usually not even precisely defined. In the case of conspiracy myths surrounding September 11, it is possible to disprove individual claims by demonstrating, for example, that hijacked airliners actually flew into the World Trade Center and caused structural damage and fires there. However, this will not prevent those who are convinced of a conspiracy from claiming that the buildings were nevertheless blown up or (if conclusive proof is presented that there could not have been a blow-up) that the U.S. government controlled the planes or at least ordered the hijacking.

Thus, in a discussion of a demand for shifting the burden of proof, there is no getting around the statement that a conspiracy claim without evidence is nothing but slander, a therapy without proof of efficacy is nothing but quackery – regardless of whether one can prove the opposite.

As a thought-provoking impulse, which may have a delayed effect, you can try to make the claim yourself that you own an invisible unicorn or that you regularly receive a visit from Ellis Kaut's red-haired children's book elf Pumuckl. In that case, you would have to be able to demand then, that this statement also had to be valid up to the proof of the opposite. If your counterpart then tries to prove the non-existence of Pumuckl, you can sit back and relax …

11.9 Just Because You Do Not Understand Why It Works …

Believers usually have a very far-reaching certainty in their felt truths. So for them, the crucial question is not whether their beliefs are true, but why others do not accept them. An obvious accusation against scientifically thinking people is that they are not able to understand in their mechanistic world view why a certain alternative therapy works or in which way one is telepathically connected with distant or deceased soul mates.

This is not an insanely far-fetched idea: if the mechanism of action of a new drug has been clarified at the molecular level and confirmed in an animal model, and if it has then been shown in a Phase I clinical trial on healthy individuals that the active ingredient is harmless and reaches the point in the body where it is supposed to act, then a Phase II trial with a few hundred patients and a Phase III trial with a few thousand patients are sufficient to apply for approval. Much more information is included in the applications for approval, but the studies themselves are initially only expected to deliver a statistically "significant" result – i.e. a difference between treated patients and placebo patients that would occur by chance in only one in 20 cases if the drug were completely ineffective.[5] Unless problems arise, the efficacy itself is often not systematically checked for a long time afterwards. Homeopaths could easily present two (possibly even methodically relatively well done) studies showing a statistically significant effect of homeopathic high potencies, i.e. of sugar globules completely free of active ingredients. Similar is the case with parapsychological studies showing effects such as telepathy. Nevertheless, this cannot be taken as proof of the effectiveness of these high potencies or of the existence of telepathy. So is there a double standard after all? Are homeopathy and parapsychological effects only rejected because it is not (yet) known how they work?

First of all, it must be stated that the study situation in these examples is not really comparable. Homeopaths and parapsychologists neglect the large number of negative or methodologically flawed studies that still exist and of which one can often only estimate how many will never be published. If five out of 100 studies deliver a statistically "significant" result, then that is exactly what would be expected by pure chance if there is no effect at all. However, studies for drug approval must be registered before they begin, so it is not possible to hide other studies with negative results.

But there is also a good reason for assigning a different value to laboratory-tested mechanisms of action than to a "proof of effect" in humans. As already explained in "He who heals is right", there are a large number of interfering factors in experiments on humans which can only be controlled with great effort – and these experiments can only ever be repeated to a limited extent.

---

[5] If two groups of test subjects do not differ systematically, the examined characteristics of the individual subjects (for example, the duration of an illness after the start of treatment) will nevertheless differ to some extent due to chance. As a result, the calculated mean values in the two groups may also differ somewhat. However, larger deviations of the mean values will be less likely than small ones. These probabilities can be calculated. A deviation in the collected data that is so large that, if there is no true effect, it should occur, purely because of chance, less frequently than in every 20th case, is called significant. In this case, one often assumes that the variation is probably not merely random, that is, that the treatment is actually better in one group than in the other.

In the case of laboratory results, the transferability to humans must always be checked, but the reliability of the data itself can be raised to an incomparably higher level. There is therefore a considerable difference between whether a study is simply intended to show that a well-understood effect that can be clearly demonstrated in the laboratory still works in the complex overall human system, or whether an effect is claimed solely on the basis of error-prone testing on an inevitably limited number of people.

With homeopathy and parapsychology it comes however still much worse: These are not only not confirmed by established results of the laboratory sciences physics and chemistry – they stand in a direct and doubtless contradiction to it. If the ideas of homeopathy were true, then central results of physics would be, as the recently deceased Berlin professor Martin Lambeck put it, *"false or grossly incomplete"* [25]. Lambeck regularly referred to the considerable number of Nobel Prizes not only in medicine, but also in chemistry and physics, which could be won if one could really prove that many alternative medical procedures have an effect beyond the placebo effect.

So it is not a matter of not knowing why something supposedly works – it is a matter of knowing with a very high degree of reliability that it cannot work. The confidence in these fundamental findings of the natural sciences will of course not remain unchallenged in a discussion with a believer. But maybe the cautious argumentation of Martin Lambeck actually helps: Of course it is conceivable in principle (as discussed in Sect. 11.5) that all physics is wrong – but when will the homeopaths finally deliver real evidence and collect their many Nobel Prizes?

11.10   The Truth Lies in the Middle

That the truth in conflicts often lies in the middle, or that there may be no objective truth to be found at all, is something we have usually already learned in childhood. In journalism, this is usually reflected in the effort to give all those involved in a dispute an equal voice. This does not only seem to be an imperative of fairness – it should also give readers, listeners or viewers the opportunity to absorb a broad spectrum of information. But this immediately leads to the problem of this supposed fairness: What if the information presented by one side is simply wrong? In this case, it is irrelevant whether the false facts are the result of deliberate disinformation, ideological delusion or a simple error.

It is not the task of television viewers or newspaper readers to investigate for themselves which of the claims presented in a discussion corresponds to the facts and which is distorted or a delusional fantasy. That would actually be the original task of the journalists who create such content. Nevertheless, time and again we find talk shows in which homeopaths, vaccination opponents or pandemic deniers are confronted with serious medical doctors on an equal footing, climatologists are supposed to discuss with climate change deniers or natural scientists with mystics. And while talk shows are – quite honestly – primarily entertainment programs, this phenomenon called "false balance" can also be found in seemingly reputable news formats. For example, as recently as October 2020 – with infections already massively on the rise – renowned epidemiologist Ulrich Mansmann had to discuss whether the pandemic was already over with Sucharit Bhakdi, a retiree who had long since slipped out of serious science, on Deutsche Welle [26]. The same constellation had been interviewed shortly before in the online magazine Cicero under the headline *"Two epidemiologists, two opinions"* [27].

The astronomer Florian Freistetter explains in a blog article why he is not available for such appearances:

> For political questions like "Is the new government good for the country?" or "Do we need tax reform?" there is no clear answer. These are indeed questions that can and must be discussed. […] But when it comes to topics like homeopathy, spiritual healing or the like, you don't have to ask yourself, "Is this all superstition?" One does not have to ask oneself, "Does homeopathy work?" or "Can astrology foresee our destiny?". Or rather, one can ask these questions, of course. But one can immediately give the correct answers (in these cases: Yes, No, No). [28]

Among the members of the science cabaret Science Busters, to which Freistetter also belongs, this is undisputed, as Science Busters protagonist Martin Puntigam points out:

> We as Science Busters no longer go into discussions if esotericists etc. are also invited. This only ennobles the counterpart and creates the appearance that it is "only about opinions". We do not discuss questions that are already answered by science.

And the physicist Florian Aigner adds [29]:

> The representatives of such refuted theses like to argue with "freedom of opinion" – but this is a gross misunderstanding. Everyone has the right to his own opinion, but no one has the right to his own facts. Of course, we must also talk about false assertions. We must not silence refuted theses – otherwise they will be woven into wild conspiracy theories all the more. But we should never present them without making it crystal clear: This is wrong.

A very similar position to the journalists responsible for such formats is taken by American politicians from the very religious southern states, who try to give the biblical creation story the same amount of time in school as evolution – and that in biology lessons. With such a supposed equal treatment, students, readers or viewers will be inclined to look for a new truth in the middle between actual truth and untruth. But how should this truth look like in the middle between medicine and spiritual healing, between astronomy and flat earth or between documentation of Nazi crimes and Holocaust denial? American physicist Bobby Henderson, responding to a discussion of creationism in school in his home state of Kansas, demanded that his own belief that the universe was created by a flying spaghetti monster should also be taught on an equal footing in school. Henderson's satire now has a worldwide following of "pastafarians" who target church privileges with demands for equal treatment.

The clear delineation between scientifically verifiable truths and unambiguous falsehoods is occasionally met with opposition from adherents of postmodernist theories of science dating back to the 1960s, who deny the existence of a reality altogether. The question of what can be known at all leads us relatively directly to the final sentence heard again and again.

11.11   There Is More Between Heaven and Earth than Your Science Can Dream of

The sentence rendered in this way is often attributed to Shakespeare, occasionally also to the legendary Chinese philosopher Laozi [30]. In fact, this sentence is questionably rephrased from Shakespeare's *Hamlet*.[6] So it is in exactly the same way a Shakespeare quote, as the immortal "He can lick my ass" from *Götz von Berlichingen* is a Goethe quote. On the one hand, it is the character in whose mouth Shakespeare put the sentence who is revealing, on the other hand, it is his situation: Prince Hamlet, freshly returned from his studies, is convinced that he has just seen a ghost who has told him that Hamlet's father has been murdered. Hamlet himself initially searches for evidence by questionable means, but then escalates into a vendetta that will lead not only him but also his entire family and his lover to their deaths.

Despite the context, which is not very worthy of imitation, the statement is not fundamentally wrong – it is just that it does not speak against scientific

---

[6] *There are more things in heaven and earth, Horatio, Than are dreamt of in our philosophy. [Later editions: your philosophy]*

thinking at all. First of all, of course, one has to realize that there are quite naturally aspects of life where it is not at all a matter of distinguishing between true and untrue from a scientific point of view. Things like love, art, music, or spirituality can be described scientifically, but in a scientific investigation about an art form, at most the investigation can be right or wrong – not the art itself. This includes storytelling, which has accompanied humanity since time immemorial and is a central part of our culture regardless of the truth of individual narratives. Nor, after all, does the value of Shakespeare's play depend on whether it truthfully tells the life story of an old Danish prince named Hamlet.

However, it is not about these topics as a rule when someone thinks that he has to emphasize that there are things that science could not dream of. Rather it is mostly used to justify claims which stand in blatant contradiction to well-established results of science. The fact that the state of science always has something provisional does not mean that there are no assured findings either. Probably, no hopefully, today's central theories of physics, the quantum theories and the theory of relativity, will eventually be replaced by new, more comprehensive concepts. But these new concepts must give the same results in practically all subjects experimentally accessible today as our current theories, because by a new theory the reality does not become different and the experiments will not have different results. Also the quantum theories and the theory of relativity do not yield different results on things which could be measured at the time of classical mechanics, than classical mechanics itself does.

So while nature is unchanging, it is our descriptions of it that are evolving, that are necessarily incomplete and provisional. The insight into this incompleteness and provisionality of our knowledge is not a criticism of science, but the precondition for being able to do science at all. This provisionality, however, does not justify filling in the unknown with arbitrary, untested fantasy creations and ascribing to them a claim to truth as facts, for example as an effective remedy. Rather, anyone who makes a claim about the unknown is under an obligation to provide evidence for it.

So, if one discusses with someone with whom this makes any sense at all, then it should at least be made clear that not knowing means nothing more than not knowing and that it can by no means be used as evidence for any placeholder truths. That one finds no explanation for an unknown observation in the sky (yet), proves neither that it is an extraterrestrial spaceship nor that it is pure imagination. The cause of this observation is simply unknown. Of course, one can also invent stories about it – but then, one must not confuse them with facts.

Isn't this enough? Just this world? Just this beautiful, complex, wonderfully unfathomable, natural world? How does it so fail to hold our attention that we have to diminish it with the invention of cheap, man-made myths and monsters? (Tim Minchin, Storm)

References

1. Schröder K (2016) Schwermetallvergiftungen mit Quecksilber und Blei bei "Ayurveda-Touristen" in Sri Lanka. Dissertation, Universität Hamburg
2. Niedersächsisches Landesamt für Verbraucherschutz und Lebensmittelsicherheit (2013) Untersuchung von Mutterkornalkaloiden in Getreideerzeugnissen. https://www.laves.niedersachsen.de/lebensmittel/rueckstaende_verunreingungen/untersuchung-von-mutterkornalkaloiden-in-getreideerzeugnissen-130616.html. Accessed on: 20. Jan. 2021
3. Ökolandbau.de (2019) Bedenkliche Pflanzeninhaltsstoffe vermeiden. https://www.oekolandbau.de/verarbeitung/produktion/qualitaetssicherung/rueckstaende/unerwuenschte-stoffe-im-lebensmittel/. Accessed on: 20. Jan. 2021
4. Govinda K (2012) Quanten-Yoga. Irisiana, München
5. Warnke U (2017) Quantenphilosophie und Spiritualität. Goldmann, München
6. Zimmerli E (2000) Quantenphysik und Bewusstseinssprung. http://www.holoenergetic.com/TX-qm-bw.htm. Accessed on: 2. Jan. 2021
7. Micali D (2020) Was mich faszinierte. https://www.danielmicali.de/FASZINATION. Accessed on: 2. Jan. 2021
8. Tenzer A (2010) Zitate von C.G. Jung. https://www.psp-tao.de/zitate/autor/CG_Jung/66. Accessed on: 2. Jan. 2021
9. Wassenberg S (2016) Biophotonen, wat is het, hoe werkt het? http://www.biolicht.nl/Biophotonen/. Accessed on: 20. Jan. 2021
10. Baier GI (2020) QuantenHeilung. https://www.gib-werte.de/quantenheilung-2-2/. Accessed on: 20. Jan. 2021
11. Klippstein N (2018) Haben unsere Gedanken und Gefühle Auswirkungen auf die Erde? http://www.nils-klippstein.de/phantasiereisen/haben-gedanken-auswirkungen/. Accessed on: 20. Jan. 2021
12. Aigner F (2020) Die Schwerkraft ist kein Bauchgefühl: Eine Liebeserklärung an die Wissenschaft. Brandstätter, Wien
13. McIntyre L (2020) Wir lieben Wissenschaft. Springer, Heidelberg
14. Herzog N (2020) Wie funktioniert die eigentlich, die Wissenschaft? https://scilogs.spektrum.de/thinky-brain/wie-funktioniert-die-eigentlich-diese-wissenschaft/. Accessed on: 2. Jan. 2021
15. Büsching F (2016) Was ist eigentlich Wissenschaft? https://www.youtube.com/watch?v=m-O-knYDlFo. Accessed on: 2. Jan. 2021

16. Montasser K (2018) Wie funktioniert Wissenschaft? In 150 Sekunden erklärt. https://www.youtube.com/watch?v=Rso98FjDPQc. Accessed on: 2. Jan. 2021
17. Transparency International (2017) Hat Monsanto Wissenschaftler gekauft? https://www.transparency.de/aktuelles/detail/article/hat-monsanto-wissenschaftler-gekauft/. Accessed on: 20. Jan. 2021
18. Reske V (2018) Darum solltet ihr nicht jeder Studie glauben. https://www1.wdr.de/wissen/wissenschaftliche-studien-100.html. Accessed on: 20. Jan. 2021
19. Kreiß C (2018) Die gekaufte Wissenschaft. https://www.sueddeutsche.de/wissen/forschungspolitik-die-gekaufte-wissenschaft-1.3875533. Accessed on: 20. Jan. 2021
20. Hagmaier B (2020) Publikationen. https://www.leuphana.de/portale/unesco-chair/publikationen.html. Accessed on: 20. Jan. 2021
21. Greenpeace (2020) Forschung für den Schutz der Hohen See. https://umweltstiftung-greenpeace.de/meeresforschung-hochseeschutz/. Accessed on: 20. Jan. 2021
22. Statistisches Bundesamt (2020) Bildung und Kultur – Finanzen der Hochschulen 2018 Fachserie 11 Reihe 4.5, Statistisches Bundesamt, Wiesbaden
23. Aulelah I (2019) Homöopathie: Kritikerin erhält Unterlassungsforderung von Globuli-Hersteller. https://www.medical-tribune.de/meinung-und-dialog/artikel/homoeopathie-kritikerin-erhaelt-unterlassungsforderung-von-globuli-hersteller/. Accessed on: 20. Jan. 2021
24. Lubbadeh J (2016) Schmutzige Methoden der sanften Medizin. https://www.sueddeutsche.de/wissen/homoeopathie-lobby-im-netz-schmutzige-methoden-der-sanften-medizin-1.1397617-0. Accessed on: 20. Jan. 2021
25. Lambeck M (2003) Irrt die Physik? Beck, München
26. Gerhäusser T (2020) Mansmann vs. Bhakdi: Corona schon vorbei? | DW Nachrichten. https://www.youtube.com/watch?v=YWOLsC31grI. Accessed on: 20. Jan. 2021
27. Cicero: Haben wir angemessen auf Covid-19 reagiert? https://www.cicero.de/innenpolitik/covid-epidemiologen-virus-bhakdi-mansmann-masken-streitgespraech. Accessed on: 20. Jan. 2021
28. Freistetter F (2018) Warum ich in Talk Shows nicht über Esoterik diskutiere. https://scienceblogs.de/astrodicticum-simplex/2018/03/13/warum-ich-in-talk-shows-nicht-ueber-esoterik-diskutiere/. Accessed on: 20. Jan. 2021
29. Aigner F (2021) Die Wahrheit liegt nicht in der Mitte. https://futurezone.at/meinung/die-wahrheit-liegt-nicht-in-der-mitte/401150706. Accessed on: 20. Jan. 2021
30. Schefter T (2020) Zitat zum Thema: Ahnungslosigkeit. https://www.aphorismen.de/zitat/85536. Accessed on: 26. Dez. 2020

12

Practical Tips

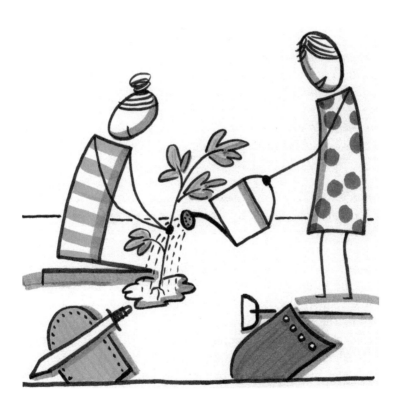

© The Author(s), under exclusive license to Springer-Verlag GmbH,
DE, part of Springer Nature 2022
H. G. Hümmler, U. Schiesser, *Fact and Prejudice*,
https://doi.org/10.1007/978-3-662-66032-4_12

If you expected a few simple rules to convince every esoteric, conspiracy believer or alternative medicine supporter of scientific thinking, then we have probably disappointed you with this book. The truth is: such discussions are not easy, and there is no sure formula that leads to success. As we have seen, there is not even a simple answer as to what can actually be considered success.

Nevertheless, there are of course always sensible attempts to summarize recommendations for discussions with believers briefly and succinctly – knowing that this can only ever do justice to a small part of the complexity of the problem. The American psychologist Michael Shermer has formulated a rather general approach in *Scientific American* as a way of dealing with the COVID pandemic and the end of the Trump era:

> If corrective facts only make matters worse, what can we do to convince people of the error of their beliefs? From my experience,

1. *keep emotions out of the exchange,*
2. *discuss, don't attack (no ad hominem and no ad Hitlerum),*
3. *listen carefully and try to articulate the other position accurately,*
4. *show respect,*
5. *acknowledge that you understand why someone might hold that opinion, and*
6. *try to show how changing facts does not necessarily mean changing worldviews.*

> These strategies may not always work to change people's minds, but now that the nation has just been put through a political fact-check wringer, they may help reduce unnecessary divisiveness.

One can argue about the general applicability of some points (emotion, for example, is also a sign of authenticity), others, such as avoiding Nazi comparisons, should actually always be a good idea if one wants to have a meaningful conversation. The sixth point in particular is exciting, though, because it is an attempt to deal with the fact that, as Chap. 2 has shown, it is so insanely difficult to break away from a worldview once accepted. A clear separation between ultimately indisputable, but in principle also value-neutral facts on the one hand and political or societal values on the other may actually help to stay in the conversation.

Despite the obvious limitations of such simplistic advice, we will try below to summarize an essence of what we have gathered in this book in short, simple statements.

12.1   Have Realistic Expectations!

The idea that you can persuade esotericists or conspiracy believers of the truth is almost a guarantee to be disappointed. In the previous chapters we have learned about a number of mechanisms that make it extremely difficult for all of us to let go of such belief systems. This is not a sign of stupidity or obduracy, but simply a part of being human. Science is characterized by helping us to repeatedly question such thought patterns ourselves or to have them questioned by others – provided that we want to do so.

But we have also seen that such lofty goals are not a necessary condition for a discussion to remain meaningful. In some circumstances, one is not discussing for the person with whom one is discussing at all, but for listeners or fellow readers. Perhaps one can shake a firmly established belief system a bit, sow a first seed of doubt, let a first breath of fresh air into a previously closed thought bubble. The success in this case will be seen much later, maybe not even by oneself. Perhaps it can be made clear that skeptics and scientists are not cold-hearted monsters, but people with feelings who also want their children to grow up healthy in a world worth living in. Perhaps the goal is simply to achieve a little more goodwill and understanding – but perhaps also to set a clear sign or a clear boundary when a person in need of protection or the functioning of democracy is in danger.

12.2   Do Not Let Yourself Be Demotivated!

Realistic goals are already a good prerequisite for not getting discouraged if you cannot convince your counterpart of the importance and reliability of scientific thinking. However, realism does not always protect you from disappointment. Sometimes you may also be met with hostility from the listeners and readers for whom you are actually conducting a discussion. When partners or close family members sink down the rabbit hole of conspiracy belief, it may also be of little comfort to have taken a stand.

However, you are not responsible for what another person believes.

In some circumstances, you have already accomplished a great deal, perhaps the maximum, by the time the person in question is even talking to you. You may be the last person outside the bubble of believers with whom a meaningful conversation is even possible. Perhaps you manage to at least offer information that would otherwise not reach the person in question at all, in a sober and deliberately time-limited exchange. Perhaps you can occasionally break through the entrenched patterns of argumentation by using humor and seemingly paradoxical objections. Perhaps you can maintain a cordial relationship despite everything by at least temporarily leaving out the subject of the dispute. Perhaps at some point, when serious doubts arise and a transformation becomes possible, you can be an anchor back into real life.

As long as you don't become a troll yourself who – mired in cynicism – keeps the discussion boiling just for the sake of arguing, you can't actually do that much wrong.

12.3 Have the Courage to Object!

Anyone who spreads objectively false information that is not just trivial entertainment, but has real, possibly harmful consequences, deserves to be contradicted. With this contradiction you help yourself not to be condemned to inaction, which you may regret later. You help listeners and fellow readers not to accept false claims as perceived truths at some point, because they have always remained unchallenged. But it also helps the person spreading the false claims, because they can otherwise chalk up the lack of contradiction as confirmation and miss a chance to challenge their unscientific beliefs.

This does not mean that you have to break out a wild argument with the babbling uncle at grandma's hitherto harmonious coffee table. You may remain calm and objective – in most cases, that's better anyway.

It doesn't mean that you have to get involved in talking the issue out on the spot. You can and may point out that a conspiracy myth is a conspiracy myth, and defer the discussion to another time or refer to experts.

It also doesn't mean that you have to be the hundredth to jump into the same notch when someone who has come out of the woodwork with doubts about certain vaccinations in a more science-oriented medical forum is cornered by an overwhelming majority of indignant vaccine advocates. The point is to show that dissent exists, not to shout down someone who might otherwise have been amenable to factual argumentation.

12.4 Have the Courage to Reconcile!

Whether one trusts in science as a method and thus ultimately in the human capacity for cognition or whether he believes in sinister powers or authorities from the beyond naturally determines not only one's picture of reality but also, to a certain extent, one's own value system. However, anyone who asks others about their star sign, carries rescue drops around in their handbag or cannot imagine that people have landed on the moon is not automatically "the enemy". If someone wants to have the chance later on to find their way out of such an anti-scientific belief system, the friendly, trustful contact to people who have always thought scientifically and stood by science is priceless. Of course, this applies in a very special way in the closer family, which often represents the last connection to outside their bubble for people who have become completely entangled in an irrational belief system. But it also applies among old classmates, among the parents on the playground or in the small animal breeders' club.

"Politics is not the measure of all things," was once said in the basic program of a German political youth organization. Neither is science – at least as long as it is not a matter of life and death.

12.5   Do Not Assume that Your Counterpart Lives in the Same World … Especially Not with Conspiracy Believers!

According to the very traditional theory of argumentation, one starts first of all from values and facts on which the participants agree. Then one tries to draw conclusions from this basic consensus according to the rules of logic, which prove one's own thesis. Even if this is often done automatically, it can be helpful, especially in heated discussions, to remember that a common basis is the starting point of the argument.

However, if one discusses with believers, especially with conspiracy believers, then one must sometimes realize that they live in a completely separate world and that a basic consensus as a basis for argumentation simply does not exist. For them, the existence of a world-dominating conspiracy is not the end result to be proven, but the unalterable fact at the beginning of all considerations. Let us assume that we succeed to prove unalterably to a convinced September 11 truther that the Pentagon was hit by a commercial airliner, that the Twin Towers were hit by the airplanes, and that the World Trade Center 7 building collapsed as a result of the following fires. This would not prove to him that the September 11 attacks were not staged by the U.S. government, but merely that the government used commercial aircraft to do so. For someone who believes in a world-wide conspiracy of pedophile Satanists, the fact that even a small component of such a network has never been uncovered is not proof that the conspiracy does not exist, but rather shows the power of this conspiracy over all police and judicial authorities in the world.

Against this background it should be clear that it is not very promising to try to convince such a person by logical argumentation. Here one can rather hope to create small cracks in the thinking system or to be there supporting and accompanying once a transformation process has begun.

With certain alternative medicine believers, who are simply convinced that they have the better studies on their side, the initial situation is possibly more favorable. However, one should be aware that even a large part of alternative medicine cannot do without the world-explaining belief in a big pharmaceutical conspiracy.

12.6   Don't Get Caught Up in Details!

Do not expect that people who reject scientific thinking lack factual knowledge. Adherents of irrational belief systems often spend considerable time acquiring detailed knowledge that at first glance seems to confirm their ideas.

Those who spend half their lives studying homeopathy can often easily cite a dozen studies that seem to prove the efficacy of homeopathic remedies. Those who have spent less time on the subject will not be able to spontaneously prove that not a single one of them has probative value according to the principles of medical science. Anyone who had been involved in the COVID denier scene since the spring of 2020, and who may not have been able to pursue his or her profession due to contact restrictions, usually had a long list of supposed evidence ready by the following winter that COVID-19 was a completely harmless cold, but that vaccinations and protective masks posed deadly dangers.

As an outsider, you will hardly have heard of most of the snippets of information often cited without sources, let alone be able to place them in the proper context or refute them. However, you do not have to get involved in such discussions. It is perfectly okay to refer to the relevant experts, literature or websites and to stop the discussion. If your counterpart is not satisfied with this, you can demand written evidence for the claims they have made. Those who give such litanies of details usually have the idea of being more scientific than the scientists and can be challenged to provide scientific evidence as well.

12.7   You Are Not Alone!

On the Internet, at work, or in groups of acquaintances, it's easy to get the feeling of facing a superior force of the irrational. This not only makes it difficult to discuss things: Those who feel isolated with their convictions experience a considerable emotional strain. Being in an environment that, at least according to subjective perception, represents completely contradictory ideas, creates the cognitive dissonance already described in Chap. 2.

In reality, however, as a representative of scientifically based views, one is rarely alone. Under certain circumstances, you may have like-minded people around you who simply do not speak out or even signal casual agreement to offensive believers in order to avoid conflict. If one cannot expect any assistance from this side, it is all the more sensible to actively seek argumentative, but above all also emotional support.

Other people who prefer well-founded facts to good-sounding stories can be found online, for example, on German Facebook in groups such as "Wissenschaft und Pseudogedöns", "Skeptisches Denken", "Mimikama & ZDDK" or "Aufklärung zu Homöopathen, Heilpraktikern und sonstigen Wunderheilern". Somewhat more satirical and specifically focused on conspiracy beliefs is the group "Nothing but the truth – Aufklärung über die Verschwörungsszene". Face-to-face meetings are made possible by the regional groups of the Society for the Scientific Investigation of Parasciences (GWUP) and its many international partner organizations, which are usually open to non-members, as well as, in the meantime, the events of the "Skeptics in the Pub" movement in many countries.

12.8   People Are Allowed to Think Differently!

With all the commitment to science and critical thinking, one must not forget that one does not have to enter into debate with every believer. Enduring dissenting opinions seems unpopular in today's world of social media shit-storms, but it's part of life.

A change of perspective, an attempt to put oneself in the other person's shoes, can in some cases show that an irrational belief may actually be just harmless entertainment, a comforting notion, or even a stabilizing force for a person's survival. Attacking someone's belief in a reunion with a loved one in the afterlife merely on principle does not make one friends, and in most cases it benefits no one. This self-reflection, which always requires a little distance, may be difficult for us, especially in the case of people who are particularly close to us.

Distinguishing such cases from those where we cannot remain silent because the lives, freedom or other well-being of vulnerable people are in danger is the true art of skeptical discussion. It is not for nothing that an English proverb advises us to choose our battles wisely.

Appendixes

Appendix A: Conclusion

Holm

There are simple, clear answers to every complex question – but unfortunately they are wrong. Whoever expected a simple guidebook from us, a cooking recipe to refute bullshit arguments and turn believers into skeptics, may now be disappointed. But there are no such simple answers. Getting someone to change their mind is incredibly difficult – simply because changing one's mind is difficult. As much as you may sometimes be scratching your head: There are people like us on the other side who are just as convinced they are right. I hope we have been able to give you a little encouragement that it is nevertheless worthwhile to embark on the adventure of such discussions – most of the time, anyway.

Ulrike

We will certainly be reproached for talking about understanding and toler-ance in the book, but then we we do pretty much play hardball with bullshit-ters, esoteric practitioners, homeopaths. For the comfort of all critics we would like to say that they are cordially invited to use all the described tools of persuasion also in the discussion with us and other skeptics. If in the end we agree that we will not convince each other, but have more understanding for each other's position and respect each other as human beings, then the work on this book has been worthwhile.

I end with the words of Science Buster Martin Puntigam: *"People are what they are. There are no better ones. You have to accept that you can't really change their minds. I'm not going to turn the pope into a radical left-wing atheist. But you have to try to at least talk to each other."*

Appendix B: Helpful Sources of Information

If you have to deal with alternative medicine, conspiracy myths, superstition or pseudoscientific half-truths, maybe unexpectedly, in a discussion, you cannot possibly have a good answer to all the questions and false claims you encounter. If such belief systems were always to be met on the basis of normal general education, surely not so many people would fall for them. Especially if the counterpart has been involved in this system for a long time and has spent a lot of time on it, one is often confronted with a vast amount of factual knowledge taken out of context. One cannot possible know all these alleged quotations of Werner Heisenberg, experiments on the flat earth from the nineteenth century, diaries of an admiral from the post-war period or studies on homeopathy with 20 patients. From this, in turn, believers naturally like to draw the confirmation that advocates of science have simply not informed themselves properly, accordingly cannot think for themselves and actually only have to watch the right YouTube videos or follow the right Telegram channel to also reach enlightenment.

Fortunately, there are also skeptical-scientific experts on almost all of these topics who have dealt with exactly this and critically questioned exactly these claims. Their information is for the most part freely available on the Internet as texts, podcasts or videos. Some of the more in-depth analyses have also been published in books or magazine articles. Quite predominantly the authors are also available for concrete, meaningful questions and, if necessary, can refer to other experts.

Appendix C: On Esotericism, Fringe Science and General Skeptical Topics

C.1 The GWUP, the Skeptical Center, the GWUP Blog and the *Skeptiker*

The *Gesellschaft zur wissenschaftlichen Untersuchung von Parawissenschaften* (Society for the Scientific Investigation of Parasciences, GWUP) is a German association of around 2000 scientists and interested lay people from a wide range of disciplines and backgrounds who are committed to promoting science and critical thinking. The GWUP also sees itself committed to consumer protection and the protection of democracy against fake news and conspiracy myths. Already on the homepage gwup.org one finds information (in German) about a multiplicity of fringe science, esoteric and alternative-medical claims in varying detail, depending upon the topic. In Roßdorf near Darmstadt the GWUP maintains a full-time presence at the *skeptical center* with an extensive archive of books and magazines on topics like fringe science and alternative medicine. As an information center for the press and interested citizens, the skeptical center can also establish contacts with experts on specific individual topics. The GWUP is also part of a worldwide network of similar organizations.

In addition to a presence in various social networks, the GWUP is present online primarily through the *GWUP blog* professionally managed by journalist Bernd Harder. The blog provides very up-to-date reports in German on a variety of corresponding topics, while the search function and keywords also provide an excellent overview of the trends of the past years.

The *Skeptiker*, the quarterly journal of the GWUP, offers well-founded analyses in greater depth. In the archive on gwup.org one can get an overview of the topics since the first issue in 1987 and order new issues directly. Articles from older issues can be forwarded by the Skeptical Center.

C.2 Deutscher Konsumentenbund

According to the external presentation of most consumer protection organizations, one can get the impression that the comprehensiveness of a bank consultation or the size of a food package play a far greater role there than the intentional or even well-intentioned deception of consumers and patients by swindlers, quacks and charlatans. The Deutscher Konsumentenbund (German Consumer Association, DKB), on the other hand, has repeatedly taken a clear position on the issues of pseudo-medicine, esotericism and life counseling in recent years. It is a good contact, especially when it comes to averting harm from potential future victims and, if necessary, taking legal action against dubious offers.

C.3 maiLab

The German YouTube channel *maiLab* around chemist Mai Thi Nguyen-Kim originally dedicated itself to the entertaining communication of natural sciences to a young audience. Parallel to the professionalization of the original one-woman project into a public network production with a full-time editorial staff, the examination of pseudoscience, pseudomedicine and conspiracy myths has become a growing theme at maiLab. "Get a cup of tea, friends of the sun!" and hear the lowdown on homeopathy, allegedly harmful fluoride, COVID myths, climate change and more in 15 min – breezily presented and YouTube-ready with lively video cuts.

C.4 Psiram and Sonnenstaatland

Psiram.com is an anonymously operated Internet project for the education about esotericism, religion and alternative medicine as well as conspiracy beliefs. The fact that the operators remain anonymous is criticized again and again. It is however simply a reaction to the fact that many bloggers had to give up, because they were covered with absurd legal proceedings by suppliers of questionable products. Even completely futile legal threats cost time, nerves and sometimes high attorneys' fees, and not every volunteer can hold out for long. Especially against Psiram and alleged Psiram authors there have also repeatedly been death threats. Psiram also has a blog, but the core of the service is an online encyclopedia with more than 3500 entries on people, companies and concepts from the above-mentioned subject areas. Most of it is only available in German, but other languages are being built up. Due to the lack of author attribution, the articles are of course not citable, but they can be a very good overview and a starting point for further research. The articles are not always completely up to date, but carefully researched and extensively documented with sources. Psiram also has a public forum for suggestions and criticism.

Especially on the German *Reichsbürger* (who believe in the continuation of the Third Reich), state deniers and related conspiracy myths there is Sonnenstaatland.com which has some similarities to Psiram in its structure with blog, forum and anonymous operators. Sonnenstaatland, however, is more satirical, and the forum, probably the most comprehensive German-language source of information on the *Reichsbürger*, is more central to the offering here.

C.5 Scienceblogs and Scilogs

Scienceblogs and *Scilogs* are collective portals for blogs on scientific topics from different disciplines. The portals are operated by major publishers, the German

Scienceblogs by Konradin Mediengruppe, Scilogs by SpringerNature. The authors are usually scientists themselves and for the most part rather young. The blog authors are invited to these blog portals after they have usually already placed successful and high-quality blog articles elsewhere or have otherwise distinguished themselves as science communicators. Since there is no centralized editing of the individual articles, the quality and above all the comprehensibility for laymen are quite different between the blogs. However, the pre-selection guarantees a certain minimum level, and the better blogs on these portals easily surpass the science sections of major daily newspapers, not only in terms of qualification, but also in comprehensibility. In particular, *Astrodicticum Simplex* by astronomer Florian Freistetter and *Fischblog* by chemist Lars Fischer (who now also writes for *Spektrum der Wissenschaft*) are among the best that German-language science journalism has to offer in written form.

C.6 Personal Projects

Mikhail Lemeshko is a young professor of theoretical physics at IST Austria in Klosterneuburg near Vienna. Scientifically, he deals with quantum phenomena in many-body systems, precisely an area that is particularly often misunderstood by laymen and particularly often distorted by charlatans. On the side, he publishes short, easy-to-understand and humorous explanatory videos on the YouTube channel *"Prof. Lemeshko"* about correct and misunderstood physics, but also about conspiracy claims and the question of what it actually means to be a scientist.

The majority of the *Nachgefragt podcast* by physicist Michaela Voth does not deal with physics topics, but rather with a broad spectrum of skeptical questions, most of which are highly relevant to society. The podcast episodes each consist of individual, detailed interviews with experts, some of whom are still quite unknown but very competent.

Quantenquark.com is the blog of Holm Gero Hümmler. Originally created as a companion project to the book *Relativer Quantenquark* (Relative Quantum Nonsense), it now covers, besides pseudophysics, conspiracy myths, science denial, and popular misconceptions, for example around COVID-19 and vaccinations. The articles are mostly long and some of them associate the topics quite freely, but the search function and keywords lead to a lot of information.

Appendix D: On Alternative Medicine

D.1 The INH, Homöopedia and Susannchen

The *Informationsnetzwerk Homöopathie* (Information Network Homeopathy, INH) is a loose network of homeopathy critics from different disciplines. Starting from a first meeting in 2015, the network provides scientific information on homeopathy and participates in the public discussion. The infrastructure of the INH like the homepage netzwerk-homoeopathie.info is supported by the GWUP and the DKB. Until she turned more to her professional development again in 2020, the interview partner for this book, the former homeopathic physician Natalie Grams, was the director of the INH. She continues to be present, for example, with the column "Grams' Sprechstunde" and the podcast of the same name on the scientific background of medicine on spektrum.de.

The *Homöopedia* (homöopedia.eu) is an online encyclopedia that emerged from the INH and contains high-quality, detailed articles, supported by scientific sources, on important topics related to homeopathy. The articles might be too long and too complex as a first introduction to a topic, but with their depth and careful source citations they are very helpful in an in-depth discussion.

Susannchen braucht keine Globuli (Little Suzie doesn't need homeopathic globules, susannchen.info) as the "family site" of the INH is less scientifically oriented, but offers easily understandable, basic information on central questions about homeopathy and alternative medicine. Many articles are specifically designed to be used as discussion starters or in comment sections.

D.2 Edzard Ernst

As a professor at the University of Exeter, Edzard Ernst held the first ever chair for the study of complementary and alternative medicine. In the course of his own research he changed from a believer in homeopathy to a skeptic and became one of the most prominent critics of pseudo-medical procedures worldwide. He retired early after a dispute with Prince Charles over the use of alternative medicine procedures in health care.

Based on his research, he has an overview of the state of scientific research on a wide range of alternative medicine procedures. He summarizes this, for example, in his recent book, *Alternative Medicine: A Critical Assessment of 150 Modalities* (Springer, 2019). On his blog edzardernst.com (in English), he reports on current research results on a wide variety of therapeutic procedures and places the respective new studies in the general research context. Especially when confronted with a lesser known procedure (Tuina, leech therapy, herbs against COVID …), Edzard Ernst's books and blog offer an almost inexhaustible treasure trove of background knowledge.

D.3 Cochrane and Medizin Transparent

Medizin Transparent is a German language Internet portal operated by the Austrian University of Krems in conjunction with the international scientific network *Cochrane,* funded by the Republic of Austria. The aim is to place health-related claims from the media, advertising and the Internet, which are often based on individual study results presented as sensational, in the overall context of the respective body of scientific knowledge. The topics cover, besides alternative procedures, also results from evidence based medicine and for example questions of nutrition.

The articles usually start with a clear question ("Is therapy X effective to achieve Y?"), followed by a clear answer, which characteristically often is: "Scientific evidence is lacking." This is followed by a more detailed article describing both the claim under investigation and the evaluation of it. Finally, the studies used are described in more detail and all claims are supported by scientific sources. The selection of topics on medizin-transparent.at is mostly based on the current news situation, but the search function and the topic overview can also be used to find targeted information on specific procedures. Due to the comprehensible, clear presentation and the scientific sources, the articles can be helpful in a wide variety of discussions on medical issues.

A thematically similar project of Cochrane Germany that is less focused on current news topics is wissenwaswirkt.org. Thus, it is less of a medical fact checker; however, the articles offer a similar structure with a short summary at the beginning, main article, and detailed sources. Cochrane publishes similar evalutations of scientific studies based on the current state of knowledge also on its homepage cochrane.de, which is rather for an expert audience.

D.4 MedWatch and IGeL-Monitor

MedWatch is a non-profit, donation-funded research portal about dangerous and dubious health claims and was awarded the German federal prize for consumer protection in 2020. The range of topics is not limited to typical alternative medicine, but also includes, for example, "individual health services" (IGeL) offered by physicians but not paid for by health insurance companies or cases of impurities in medicines. Since the project has only been in existence since 2017, it does not have the thematic breadth of, for example, *Medizin Transparent*, but with its more journalistic approach it can not only present the scientific state of knowledge, but also includes, for example, information on the background of the providers or on ongoing health policy discussions.

With regard to individual health services, MedWatch also likes to refer to the *IgeL Monitor*, which systematically classifies and evaluates such additional services offered by physicians on the basis of scientific studies. These include typical alternative medical procedures such as Bach flower therapy, but also various screening tests or cosmetic procedures such as tattoo removal. Due to the careful source references, this portal is also particularly suitable when a discussion goes into scientific detail.

D.5 Websites of Public Authorities

Particularly on health topics, reliable information that can be referred to can also be found on the websites of the relevant authorities – and the comprehensibility and design of the information on these sites has become increasingly better in recent years.

In Germany, the *Bundeszentrale für gesundheitliche Aufklärung* (Federal Center for Health Education, BzgA) is responsible for communicating health issues to the general population. It became known primarily in the 1990s for its AIDS education campaigns. At bzga.de you will find mainly longer-running campaigns on prevention and common diseases, but also information on current topics.

The *Robert Koch Institut* (RKI) is Germany's national public health institute and is primarily responsible for combating infectious diseases and analyzing health trends in the population. In the COVID pandemic, the website rki.de which was originally aimed primarily at a specialist audience, has become a popular source of information for the general public. It is especially helpful for people interested in science and for high-level discussions.

Less in the public eye than the RKI is the *Paul Ehrlich Institut* (PEI), which is responsible for the supervision of vaccines and biomedical drugs. The website pei.de is therefore even more focused on a specialist audience, but can also provide helpful information for discussions on vaccination topics.

What one will unfortunately look for in vain on all these pages, is critical attention to alternative medicine.

Appendix E: On Conspiracy Myths and Fake News

E.1 Mimikama

The site mimikama.at is run by an Austrian "Verein zur Aufklärung über Internetmissbrauch" (Association for Information on Internet Abuse) which is funded by donations and previously advertising on its website. The name of the associated Facebook page "Think first – then click" still indicates that the original focus of the offer was on Internet fraud and subscription traps. In the meantime, however, conspiracy myths and politically motivated disinformation (fake news) have been added as core topics, as have accidental false news.

For the German-speaking Internet, Mimikama has become the first port of call for questioning dubious news, from vaccination scares about alleged sightings of mythical creatures to false quotes from politicians and celebrities. The site sometimes appears rather confusing at first glance, but the scope of the available information and the solidity of the research are actually beyond compare.

E.2 Correctiv and ARD Faktenfinder

In addition to Mimikama, there are several other formats in the German-speaking world that are dedicated to fact-checking current news. The best known is probably the non-profit research center *Correctiv*, which also carries out fact checks for Facebook. The evaluations of current reports and allegations appear predominantly on their own page correctiv.org.

On the German public news media page tagesschau.de you can find articles on current reports in the *ARD Faktenfinder* section, but for the most part they do not follow the typical true-false format of other fact checks, but rather represent normal editorial text contributions.

E.3 Volksverpetzer

The *Volksverpetzer* is originally a clearly left-leaning political blog, which over the past few years has shifted its focus to dealing with far-right propaganda, fake news and conspiracy myths, and in the COVID pandemic has become one of the most important information portals about the alternative facts scene. In addition to its focus on content, the Volksverpetzer also distinguishes itself from a typical political blog through very solid research and documentation of the sources used.

E.4 Hoaxilla

In this German podcast, psychologist Alexander Waschkau and cultural scientist Alexa Waschkau take a scientific look at all kinds of mysterious stories, from urban legends to conspiracy myths to curiosities from history and space travel. In addition to a sober look at the facts, the social and cultural significance of the events under consideration and the stories that revolve around them come up. The regular episodes, of which 267 had already been published by the end of 2020, always deal in detail with a key topic, so that the archive at hoaxilla.com can now refer to a considerable spectrum of topics. These episodes are usually conducted by the two of them alone, but sometimes with the help of experts. In addition, there is a whole series of special episodes, mostly in interview form.

In the 2020 COVID pandemic, the talk format *Ferngespräch* with TV comedian Tommy Krappweis, Hoaxilla, author Holm Gero Hümmler and others was then created as a video stream on twitch.tv of which past episodes can still be seen on YouTube. Audio recordings of all *Ferngespräch* episodes appear as podcast specials on Hoaxilla. For 2022 Hoaxilla is also planning an animation series on television.

E.5 Snopes

Snopes.com describes itself as the "the internet's go-to source for discerning what is true and what is total nonsense", and at least for the English-speaking world, this immodest self-assessment is probably true. Founded back in the mid-1990s as an online encyclopedia for urban legends, the portal has become the most important American fact checker, especially for political fake news, even before the Trump era. The site, which is still run by its founder as a private company, has repeatedly been certified by other organizations as having great objectivity and political neutrality. Similar to Mimikama, the readership is called upon to help with the research by sending in questions, but also their own findings.

Another important fact-checking site for the U.S. is politifact.com, run by the nonprofit journalism school Poynter Institute. With a brief true-false classification at the beginning, followed by more detailed analysis with sources, the format of the articles is very similar to Snopes. Charming is the Politifact *Truth-o-Meter*, which briefly summarizes the truth content of the news story under investigation: The wildest rumors receive a rating of "Pants on fire."

E.6 Metabunk

While the typical fact-checking sites are primarily concerned with false news, metabunk.org focuses on research into conspiracy allegations. The portal is not set up as a classic information website or blog, but uses relatively old-fashioned forum software with sub-forums for various discussion topics. The initiator, the British-American author Mick West, thus deliberately relies on interaction and joint research with his numerous forum members.

If you are unfamiliar with such forums or have already forgotten they existed, this type of presentation does take some getting used to. However, the forums are well moderated, so that there are relatively few content-less queries or comments between posts that really contain substantial information. At the same time, especially on typical American conspiracy myths such as 9/11, UFO sightings, the flat earth, or chemtrails, there is such thorough research, even on detailed questions, as is rarely found in summary articles or even in books.

Appendix F: On Religious Questions

Whoever hears the word "cult" probably thinks of Scientology and Bhagwan, of mass suicides and people who proselytize in pedestrian zones. However, counseling centers in this field deal with much broader phenomena. Basically, they are concerned with all areas in which spirituality and religion do not serve to strengthen people, but are misused for the interests of a community or a guru. Experts on spiritual communities also avoid the term "cult" because it is one-dimensional and discriminatory. However, there are indeed individuals and groups that create cult-like structures, there are destructive group dynamics and methods of manipulation and brainwashing. They are often subtle and inconspicuous and can rarely be prosecuted. The focal points of our work are esotericism, guru movements, radical and extremist ideologies, dubious offers from the coaching, education and seminar sectors, conspiracy myths, occultism, spiritual and miracle healings, dropout communities, "Freemen"/sovereign citizens/*Reichsbürger*, multi-level marketing and pyramid schemes. What these different topics have in common is that their adherents sometimes change in ways that appear "cult-like" to others after contact with the respective group or worldview. For example, they fanatically promote the ideology/product, invest time and money in it, break off old contacts and change in a negative way. Sometimes there is unhealthy dependence on one person. Only a few experts deal with the (group) psychological mechanisms of these communities and even fewer offer therapeutic support for those affected and their relatives.

In addition to knowledge about the mechanisms, the following counseling centers also have knowledge about frequently mentioned persons, movements, procedures and products. In case of doubt, you can ask whether a product or method is scientifically based or originates from the esoteric field, whether negative experiences have already been reported about a certain offer, and how to deal with relatives who find themselves under the influence of a problematic group or guru. If you yourself have had negative experiences with an offer from this field, a report about it can be useful for later inquiries. It might be helpful for you to talk to someone if you have doubts about whether a community is good for you, or if you have withdrawn after negative experiences and want to process and understand what you went through.

In most cases, the websites of these agencies are less up-to-date and comprehensive. Primarily checklists and articles of a general nature can be found. Lists of problematic groups and individuals are rare, as efforts are made to avoid generalizations and legal disputes. Personal counseling is offered preferentially.

F.1 State-Funded Counseling Centers in the German-Speaking Countries

Bundesstelle für Sektenfragen (Austria)
Wollzeile 12/2/19
A-1010 Wien
Tel.: +43 1513 04 60
bundesstelle@sektenfragen.at
www.bundesstelle-sektenfragen.at
SektenInfo Berlin (Germany)
Senatsverwaltung für Bildung, Jugend und Familie
Bernhard-Weiß-Str. 6
D-10178 Berlin
+49 30 90227–5574
post@senbjf.berlin.de
www.berlin.de/sen/jugend/familie-und-kinder/sekteninfo-berlin/
Sekten-Info NRW (Germany)
Rottstraße 24
D-45127 Essen

Tel: +49 201 23 46 46
kontakt@sekten-info-nrw.de
https://sekten-info-nrw.de
Zebra (Germany)
BW Zentrale Beratungsstelle für Weltanschauungsfragen
Esoterik- und Religionsinfo BW e.V.
Gartenstr.15
D-79098 Freiburg
Tel.: +49 761 48 89 82 96
info@zebra-bw.de
https://zebra-bw.de
infoSekta (Switzerland)
Fachstelle für Sektenfragen
Streulistrasse 28
CH-8032 Zürich
Tel: +41 44 454 80 80
info@infosekta.ch
www.infosekta.ch

F.2 Church-Run Counseling Centers

Out of respect for religious freedom and in order not to appear intolerant and discriminatory, government institutions tend to show restraint in the area of spirituality and religion. Expertise in the field of so-called cults therefore lies in large part with the Catholic and Protestant churches.

Evangelische Zentralstelle für Weltanschauungsfragen (Germany)
Auguststraße 80
D-10117 Berlin
Tel.: +49 30 28395–211
kbinfo@ezw-berlin.de
www.ezw-berlin.de
Kirche im Dialog – Bereich Weltanschauungsfragen (Austria)
Stephansplatz 4/Stiege 7/1. Stock
A-1010 Wien
Tel: +43 1 51552–3384
rfw@edw.or.at
www.weltanschauungsfragen.at

Evangelische Informationsstelle Kirchen – Sekten – Religionen (Switzerland)
Wettsteinweg 9
CH-8630 Rüti ZH
Tel.: +41 55 260 30 80
info@relinfo.ch
www.relinfo.ch